WITHDRAWN

Learning to Speak Alzheimer's

Learning to Speak
Alzheimer's

A Groundbreaking Approach for
Everyone Dealing with the Disease

■ ■ ■

Joanne Koenig Coste

HOUGHTON MIFFLIN COMPANY

BOSTON   NEW YORK

2003

For information about permission to reproduce selections
from this book, write to Permissions, Houghton Mifflin Company,
215 Park Avenue South, New York, New York 10003.

Visit our Web site: www.houghtonmifflinbooks.com.

Library of Congress Cataloging-in-Publication Data
Coste, Joanne Koenig.
Learning to speak Alzheimer's : a groundbreaking approach
for everyone dealing with the disease / Joanne Koenig Coste.
p.   cm.
Includes index.
ISBN 0-618-22125-5
1. Alzheimer's disease—Patients—Care—Popular works.
2. Alzheimer's disease—Patients—Rehabilitation—Popular
works. 3. Caregivers—Popular works. I. Title.
RC523.2.C67 2003
362.1'96831—dc21   2003051141

Printed in the United States of America

Book design by Victoria Hartman

MP 10 9 8 7 6 5 4 3 2 1

To TEDDIE, my beloved husband,
who provided the structural and emotional space
to pen these pages, along with reams of computer
paper, Massenet and Mozart in the background,
silence when necessary, breakfast in bed, lectures as
needed, and love.

And to PAUL RAIA, a.k.a. "Dr. Know,"
who for more than two decades has led thousands
of families to more positive and productive places
with his witty style, habilitative wisdom, and
compassionate advice.

Acknowledgments

This book has taken a very long time to research and write. My ideas for living through the process of Alzheimer's disease, and doing so with an occasional smile, have been enriched by the feelings expressed by the patients and care partners I have worked with over the past three decades. My suggestions have been validated by a multitude of professionals who daily make life kinder for this very special fellowship of memory-impaired adults and those who love them.

I've designed the book to underscore my philosophy of living in the patients' world — of reaching them through their remaining emotions, and, when words fail, "listening" to their eyes. I have attempted to capture the feelings of those whose verbal language is failing in my poems at the opening of each chapter. I hope this will assist the reader in comprehending the emotion and the remaining cognition behind the loss of memories.

I am deeply grateful to my children, Scott, Wendy, Kristen, and Jason, who have always been the root of my strength and dearly loved. Many thanks also to Mimi and Grampy, who said, "Of course you can"; to Todd, for his hugs and warm words; to Garrett, who learned to say "Just a minute and I'll get her" as part of his daily routine; and to my precious darlings, Shay, GG, Jamie, Ty, and Hunter, whose faces beam at me from a desktop photo and keep me centered.

From deep within my heart I thank Nancy Stone Hindlian and Linda Gibson, who have taught me a deeper and more profound meaning of the word "sister." To Carrie Jochelson, Dr. Dilar Acar, Dr. Jeanne

Richard, and Cheryl Weinstein—thank you for teaching me how to listen to myself. I offer this book up to heaven as well—to Helen Stone and Paul Wilson for snapshots of life reflected through loving eyes.

I joyfully acknowledge Muriel Baum, Dick Blinn, Jerry Flaherty, Paul McCarty, Walter Ohanian, Dan O'Leary, Dr. Harold Schiff, Dr. Dennis Selkoe, Mike Splaine, Dr. Marrott Sinex, Marilyn Stasonis, and a myriad of other health care professionals who were there beside me in the earliest days of pioneering compassionate best-practice efforts for those with Alzheimer's disease. Thanks also to Mark Ailinger and Kate Salmon, who continue to help.

For my friends Lois Pecora, Paul Raia, and Elaine Silverio, who have sat beside me as facilitators of early-stage patient groups for many years, thanks for the sharing, the laughter, the untamed joy, and the tears. You have given unconditionally and helped thousands—how lucky I have been to share this journey with you.I must thank Laura van Dam, editor extraordinaire, for believing in this book from the beginning—her sense of what's right and her compassion go hand in hand; Erica Avery, who has made this process much smoother; Janet Silver, publisher and editor-in-chief, for standing so firmly behind this endeavor; Bridget Marmion, director of marketing, and Lori Glazer, executive director of publicity, whose support for this book has been gratifying and exhilarating; Suzanne Cope and Gracie Doyle, whose thoughts and energy in the marketing and publicity for this book have already been extraordinary; Peg Anderson, manuscript editor, who showed me wonderful new ways to be a writer; and all the other great people at Houghton Mifflin.

Thanks to Bill Patrick, who initially edited my words into a book that I'm proud to have written. To my agent, Jeff Kleinman, of Graybill and English, I offer much gratitude for sharing many joyous accomplishments and for pushing, applauding, and being there at all hours to write with me, guide me, chastise gently, and lead me on this journey into myself. You are the greatest, Jeff.

Above all, this book would not have been possible without countless patients and the care partners who have helped them. I am grateful to everyone who shared anecdotes, joys, fears, tears, and laughter with me. Each person is a part of my memory bank, and each has made my heart fuller. Thank you.

Contents

PART THREE

Beyond Habilitation

Foreword

Alzheimer's disease is one of the great scourges of old age in the twenty-first century. Devastating, irreversible, and progressive, it robs millions of older Americans of their use of language, reasoning, memory, and judgment. Alzheimer's destroys a lifetime of memories and whittles away at the core of a person's identity. It irrevocably alters the lives of families who have a member with Alzheimer's, often necessitating a painful redefinition of the primary relationship between parents and children, between husband and wife. Alzheimer's disease exacts an enormous emotional, physical, and psychological toll upon caregiving family members.

The third most costly disease after heart disease and cancer, Alzheimer's places an enormous burden on the U.S. health care system. Experts estimate that the dollar cost to the nation of caring for people with Alzheimer's was more than $100 billion in 2002, with neither Medicare nor most private health insurance providers covering the long-term care that most patients eventually need. The cost to American businesses in 2000 was more than $61 billion, with the costs of absenteeism, productivity loss, and employee replacement as a result of family caregiving consuming $36.5 billion.

In 2002, 45 percent of the National Institute on Aging (NIA) research budget was earmarked for research on Alzheimer's disease. That percentage represents a major advance over the funding level in 1975, when I became the founding director of the NIA and identified the study of Alzheimer's and other dementias as a key priority. From 1955 to 1962 I had worked at the National Institute of Mental Health, studying healthy aging and dementias full-time, and I continued to do so part-time thereafter. When I began to prioritize the research agenda at the NIA, my clinical and scientific interest in dementia contributed to the decision to promote research in Alzheimer's.

Up to that time "senility" was the popular term used to describe all the dementias. Patients, doctors, and scientists alike viewed a diagnosis of dementia with a sense of hopelessness. Their pessimism stemmed from the false belief that senility — the dementias — was an inevitable result of aging. Dementias were often presumed to be the result of cerebral arteriosclerosis (colloquially known as "hardening of the arteries"); researchers didn't recognize preventive measures for that condition until the 1970s. In that era, doctors assumed that Alzheimer's disease was a rare form of senility that began before age sixty.

The image of the senile man or woman, the traditional stereotype of old age in Western society, was translated into hesitancy on the part of social and scientific policymakers to invest in research into the basic biology of aging. The rationale was that money spent on aging research was money wasted on the decrepit and incompetent.

In 1975 the government funded only twelve grants for the study of "brain aging," totaling $700,000. But concern was building about Alzheimer's, eventually resulting in the successful mobilization of federal and private philanthropic resources. In 1979, twelve independent groups for Alzheimer's disease existed in the United States and Canada. Dr. Donald Tower, director of what was then known as the National Institute of Neurological and Communicative Disorders and Stroke, and I brought together representatives of those groups and urged them to unite.

Their consolidation constituted the beginnings of the present-day Alzheimer's Association.

Around the same time, the public began to learn about the disease through the media. Princess Yasmin Aga Khan appeared on *20/20* with Hugh Downs and spoke compassionately about her mother, the former movie actress Rita Hayworth, who was afflicted with the disease. Abigail Van Buren, of "Dear Abby" fame, also helped develop awareness of the disease through her column. And the National Institute on Aging in conjunction with the Neurology and Mental Health Institutes sponsored a symposium led by neurologists Robert Katzman and Robert Terry, along with Kathryn Bick of the Neurology Institute, that focused on Alzheimer's disease. The book that resulted from the symposium, *Alzheimer's Disease: Senile Dementia and Related Disorders* (New York: Raven Press, 1978), stimulated research in the field.

Senator Thomas Eagleton and Congressman Joseph Early supported the initial efforts to make Alzheimer's a national research priority. Today the federal government, voluntary organizations, and private industry provide support for research, public education, and critical services to people with Alzheimer's and their families. This funding has enabled scientists to make valuable progress in understanding the genetic, molecular, and cellular aspects of the basic biology and neurobiology of aging. And clinical trials are now under way to test potentially useful drugs for Alzheimer's. But until effective treatments are found, we must continue to work on behalf of the growing number of people who deal with the disease.

First we must redesign and expand Medicare to finance long-term-care services at home, in the community, and, when necessary, in nursing homes. And we need to ensure proper care at home, where 75 percent of the care for people with Alzheimer's takes place. An Alzheimer's patient requires constant care and vigilance, often for many years.

As *Learning to Speak Alzheimer's* makes clear, family members and others intimately involved in caring for patients need support in finding constructive ways to handle the inevitable stress, tension, and frustration of dealing with this extraordinarily challenging disease. Supportive professional advice is essential in the day-to-day struggles of caregivers, who constantly have to overcome their sense of helplessness as they observe the ongoing mental and physical erosion of a loved one.

Finding ways to provide such advice is in the best interest of both the government and employers. Caregivers often have to juggle home, child care, and adult caregiving responsibilities with paid employment, necessitating that they take off many hours and days from work to fulfill their obligations. The Alzheimer's Association estimates that each full-time employed caregiver of a patient with Alzheimer's loses, on average, about twenty-four days a year.

With the aging of the baby boomers, government experts estimate that the number of people diagnosed with Alzheimer's disease will dramatically increase, and costs will become unsustainable. Clearly, it is critically important to accelerate drug research and find more effective means of prevention and treatment. Our society must rise to this scientific and cultural challenge. The search for a cure has expanded in recent years through research to determine genetic and environmental factors that cause Alzheimer's. Neuroscience is making great advances, propelled by cell biology, chemistry, genomics, and imaging technology, and in the past ten years, some exciting findings have provided clues to the causes of the disease. But private as well as public investment in research must be accelerated, with more funding for drug discovery and development by academic laboratories and biotechnology companies.

As people live longer, their susceptibility to Alzheimer's disease increases. Today, for every five-year group beyond age sixty-five, the percentage of people with the disease doubles. Until a solution is found, that statistic will not change. One quarter of the population over seventy-five will continue to be stricken, and attitudes toward old age will continue to be shaped by the fear of cognitive decline.

Old age without dementia will be the medical triumph of the twenty-first century.

—Robert N. Butler, M.D.,
president and chief executive officer,
International Longevity Center—U.S.A.,
and professor of geriatrics and adult development,
Mount Sinai School of Medicine

PART ONE

Learning
about
Alzheimer's

· 1 ·

The Ticking Meter

My head feels like an old depot,
worn by time and tears.
No more locomotives passing through,
café filled with tales and baggage.
The old depot's barren now.
There has been a great brain robbery.

ONE COOL SPRING DAY in 1971, the kind that makes
New Englanders smile at each other, I was driving with my husband down the main street of a small coastal town south of
Boston. I spotted a parking space in front of our destination, a
café where we dined frequently, sharing chowder, fried clams, gi-
gantic iced teas, and dreams of the future.

I told my husband, "Look, there's a parking space. Not only
that — there's money in the meter."

"I'm glad," he murmured, seeking my eyes through his sun-
glasses. "But I think my meter is running out."

His metaphor fell on deaf ears. With a new life growing inside
me — our fourth child — I may have been unwilling to accept
his meaning.

At the time my husband's lapses in memory seemed innocuous. He might forget a neighbor's name or neglect to stop at the store or forget where the ignition was in the car, but I was clever at disregarding the hints of medical illness. After all, he frequently drove different cars as part of his advertising business, and he was so busy; keeping up with minor details was too much to expect. *The situation will improve when we move into a new house,* I told myself, or *when the children are older,* or *when someone in the medical community will listen to what I am saying.*

We moved, the children grew, and the improvement never happened. We were near financial ruin. Customers weren't calling us back; new jobs weren't coming our way. He had ever greater difficulty focusing and organizing his thoughts, sometimes rewriting ad copy he had finished the day before. Once so gentle, docile, and fun to be around, he became frustrated and angry. My mantra continued whenever I was awake: "Things will be so much better when —" When?

Our journey into the world of dementia began in 1971, when no guideposts, advocates, manuals, or support groups were available to help us. The National Alzheimer's Association would not be organized for another decade. My husband was only in his forties, and I did not believe that his forgetfulness was a natural part of aging. The children chided their father occasionally about his "absent-mindedness" but seemed to see nothing deeper. The prescription for Valium to treat his supposed "depression" was refilled many times. And sometimes my husband unwittingly doubled the dose or forgot to take it at all.

Always well dressed in the past, my handsome, athletic husband began to need help matching his suit, tie, and shirt. I started to lay out his clothes for the next day before we went to bed at night. I made sure to tell him what fun I had selecting the outfits, but I was embarrassed to be doing this task. I never mentioned it to others.

Then in 1973, a major stroke paralyzed him on one side, and I replaced the Brooks Brothers suits with sweatsuits, which he soon stained with food. The stroke took away his language ability, transforming a man who had made his living through eloquent writing into someone who had to rely entirely on words of one syllable. Neurologists and physical therapists told me not to expect any improvements in his speech though he did learn to walk again, ever so slowly, with a leg brace and a walker. Life was very hard for all of us, but it was especially horrible for my husband. He became frustrated beyond comprehension.

At times he did not seem to recognize our children or me. Sometimes he appeared thoroughly perplexed about our home. I remember him angrily rattling the doorknob in an effort to go outside but not being able to open the door. And yet I also recall his having enough of his former self that when he looked at our young baby, tears would run down his face.

His abilities continued to decline. As soon as I became the least bit comfortable with his current condition, he would take another step in the downhill progression of dementia. I felt completely overwhelmed. At times I was diapering both our youngest child and my husband. *There's no way I can do this,* I would think to myself.

Finally things came to a head. My husband kept opening the door to go outside — as if to escape from what was happening to him — and my toddler would follow him out. Soon our son started trying to open the door and walk out on his own (this was before safety devices were so readily available). I realized I had to act — proactively, positively, and immediately, before my husband and son left home and got lost. I installed a new handle higher on the door, leaving the old knob intact but disabled. My son could no longer reach the door. More incredibly to me, my husband didn't understand the concept of the new handle: he would repeatedly go over to the door, try the old knob, and think that the door was broken.

This tiny event made me realize that I could make some changes in the way we were living. I could stop walking on eggshells, in fear of what would happen next, and start making a positive difference in our surroundings and in my approach to his illness. I'm a very competitive person, and I started thinking of the entire situation as a game — a brand-new game I wanted to win. I knew I had to get suited up and be ready to play. Each daily task — eating, dressing, toileting, everything — was a new inning, a new round in this game.

I stopped making excuses for the changes in his behavior and the decline in his cognitive functions. The neurologist had told me that my husband's disease was progressive and would be fatal — and in an odd way, that knowledge helped me. It gave me the energy I needed to cope with what he and I both faced, because I knew that the situation would not go on forever.

I vowed to learn to live with this person who was inhabiting the body of the man I cherished. I had to detach myself emotionally from the man my husband used to be and live now with the man he had become. The task at hand — this minute, and every minute of every day — was to ensure my family's survival; I couldn't waste time focusing on my lot in life. I had to deal with the reality of today.

I decided not to heed the hospital social workers who told me that my husband would be "fine" if he went to live at an institution for the mentally ill or at a nursing home for the elderly, where he would be with others suffering from dementia. In that era, I did not trust that hospital and nursing-home workers would try to connect with him. And I knew that if he stayed at home, I could still reach parts of this man. A great deal of the time, his emotions seemed akin to mine. If I can reach him on an emotional level, I thought, instead of on a verbal or cognitive one, maybe life can be less threatening and frustrating for him.

I started a two-part list of issues related to his illness. Those elements that I thought could be changed, ameliorated, or implemented I put in part one. The elements that no amount of concentrated effort could ever change I listed in part two. I wrote "improved mobility" on the first list, while I relegated "return of speech" to the second. I placed "daily laughter" on the list of goals that could be implemented and "planting the garden" on the list of those that could not. Eventually my lists filled a spiral-bound notebook, with several hundred entries.

After putting into practice the ideas and goals on the first list, I found that a smile from my husband, calmness in our household, meant a win for all of us. I wanted to laugh at the end of the day, not curl up in a corner or break down in despair.

From the items in my notebook I developed five simple tenets, which I now teach to people who care for patients with Alzheimer's disease or related forms of progressive dementia such as vascular dementia, Pick's disease, and Lewybody disease. These ideas are the basis for the humanistic approach to caring that I call "habilitation." The literal meaning of habilitate is "to clothe or dress," but I use it in the sense of "to make capable," which is actually an older meaning of the word. A habilitated person with dementia can live using his or her upper limits of function, intellect, emotion, and spirit. Using the tenets of habilitation, both patients and care partners can feel successful at what they do, rather than feeling constantly weighted down. (I prefer the terms "care partner" or "habilitator" to "caregiver," which assumes less involvement on the part of the patient.)

The following are the tenets that I developed, first for my own use at home and later for the use of other patients with dementias.

1. *Make the Physical Environment Work.* Simplify the environment. Accommodate perceptual loss by eliminating distractions.

2. *Know That Communication Remains Possible.* Remember that the emotion behind failing words is far more important than the words themselves and needs to be validated. Although many losses occur with this disease, assume that the patient can still register feelings that matter.

3. *Focus Only on Remaining Skills.* Value what abilities remain. Help the patient compensate for any lost abilities without bringing them to his or her attention.

4. *Live in the Patient's World.* Never question, chastise, or try to reason with the patient. Join her in her current "place" or time, wherever that may be, and find joy with her there.
5. *Enrich the Patient's Life.* Create moments for success; eliminate possible moments of failure, and praise frequently and with sincerity. Attempt to find humor wherever possible.

These tenets require continuous examination of how the patient thinks, feels, communicates, compensates, and responds to change, emotion, and love. Improving understanding in these areas can lead to the biggest successes in treatment.

Along with my direct experience, my decades of work with professional and family care partners have shown that the habilitation approach *works.* Having worked with thousands of patients and care partners over the years, I have come to know that even people with fatal neurological illnesses still possess the innate drive to maximize their potential. After observing the success of the habilitation approach, colleagues and friends began to study and implement the tenets themselves, easing the burden of care partners, developing activities for Alzheimer's patients, studying those in long-term care, and addressing their special architectural and interior design needs. All of these researchers from varying disciplines have long believed in and studied the innate drive that remains in people with neurological diseases such as Alzheimer's. This shared belief has led to a clearer understanding of why we should continue to focus on patients' positive aspects and remaining skills.

During the years I care partnered with my husband, I clarified the tenets, and both he and I were able to succeed at living under our changed circumstances. When he died in 1976, I moved back to my parents' home with our four children, whose ages ranged from four to sixteen. I had told my parents that I wanted to stay with them just for a few weeks to figure out what I should do with the rest of my life; instead I stayed for fifteen years. The children grew up, and I bandaged cut fingers and injured spirits. They participated in Pop Warner football, Little League baseball, high school soccer, track, and championship swimming. They found friendship and love and went on to colleges and careers. Now that they are enriching the lives of others, I often wonder how they would have matured without the years of turmoil and distress, fear of the unknown, and terror of the known that they endured. Perhaps support and love for all of our family — my husband included — offset family tragedy.

After moving in with my parents, I immediately began working as a nursing assistant in a nursing home run by a local hospital. I soon became director of restorative services, which let me initiate a program to try to help several residents who had progressive dementias — and who at that time bore such lofty diagnoses as "organic" and "chronic" brain syndrome. Before long, newly admitted people wanted to be included in the program, which was based on the habilitative tenets described above. I led daily sessions with the patients, worked with the care partners at the facility, and developed a support group for spouses. I have been leading such groups continually since 1978, and this work remains a great joy in my life.

The nursing home developed a special-care unit for the patients in the program, and soon we recognized that they were doing much better cognitively than they had done before and were participating more fully in daily living activities, such as dressing and bathing. All of the patients appeared calmer, which meant that their medications could be reduced. In this unit, restraints were removed; hugs were instituted.

After successfully mentoring the staff and performing daily cognitive and supportive interactions with a population that grew to comprise more than half of the patient roster at the facility, I attempted to have this new kind of care — the habilitative approach — recognized by state and national regulatory agencies concerned with confidentiality and the right to a private diagnosis. But in the 1970s, civil libertarians and others were loath to have specific beds set aside for patients with dementias. They were concerned that such groupings would reveal the patients' diagnoses, which would be an invasion of privacy.

I was very lonely during that time. I had no one to talk to about changing the scene for cognitively impaired adults. Alzheimer's was beginning to be given as a diagnosis, even though it was treated as a brand-new discovery; but except for a few colleagues at the nursing home, no one was willing to listen to my ideas. I was so elated when I discovered John Panella at Cornell University, who was studying the impact of special programming on patients with Alzheimer's disease at a day care facility in White Plains, New York. At last I had discovered someone else who believed that we could make a difference in the lives of Alzheimer's patients.

The establishment in 1980 of the National Alzheimer's Association gave me and the growing number of concerned individuals and organizations renewed courage to fight for specialized housing and programming. By 1981 the program at the nursing home where I worked became an officially sanctioned special unit. As attempts to duplicate it popped up all over the Northeast, I became happily busy teaching and mentoring.

During the next two decades, the National Alzheimer's Association grew, with branches in every state offering family support and patient care, professional education, research opportunities, and advocacy. And as other professionals became interested in the care of people with Alzheimer's, the effort to institute habilitative settings became easier. Advocates traveled to state houses and government agencies to describe the major differences that specialized care made in the lives of Alzheimer's patients, their families, and the staff of institutions caring for them. Special-care units now exist in every region of the United States, and specific programming for people with Alzheimer's disease and the related disorders are common in adult day health, assisted-living, and retirement centers.

Still, families need to be wary of institutions that claim to offer specialized care but do little more than secure the doors. Without trained staff, ongoing education, and a habilitative philosophy of care adopted by the whole staff, the unit is not "special." Both the National Alzheimer's Association and its state chapters can help sort through the differences.

For people seeking care for patients outside the home, as well as those planning to provide care themselves, this book teaches both the habilitation philosophy and the practical techniques that make care partnering effective and enriching. It focuses primarily on the early and middle stages of Alzheimer's and other progressive dementias, when habilitative care can be most effective.

This book is divided into three parts. In Part One, to foster an understanding of Alzheimer's disease and to underscore how altered behavior relates to the changes in the brain, I present an overview of the disease in lay terms. I then discuss some of the most common issues immediately affecting people with Alzheimer's.

Part Two moves into the core idea of habilitation — creating a positive milieu in which the patient can enjoy feelings of success. I focus on basic, simple suggestions for use of leisure time and offer practical solutions for bathing, dressing, toileting, and eating independently. I include tips for communication and for dealing with negative behaviors.

Part Three discusses the need for care partners to take care of themselves and provides a summary of short- and long-term-care options most conducive to the habilitation principles.

At the end of the book, the Appendix and Further Resources provide the most practical, useful information I've been able to compile — from simple finger food suggestions to books and other reference materials to companies and dealers who specialize in materials I use in my habilitation work.

Most of the anecdotes used throughout the book are composites based on stories I have heard through the years or incidents in which I was a participant. While the dialogue is often based only on my impressionistic memory, the deeper truth contained in each vignette is real. I selected the anecdotes to show what remains in the heart and soul of the person with Alzheimer's disease or other progressive dementia, and to help care partners move into the patient's world and focus not on what is missing but on what is still there.

If you are a care partner, remember to be kind to yourself as you read through the ideas presented here. Do not try to implement all the ideas at once, since that would be overwhelming. After all, the goal of habilitation is to create a positive emotional and physical environment for the care partner as well as for the patient. Figuring out what most needs to be done at any moment makes achieving the overall goal far more manageable. Congratulate yourself on what you can do.

Seeking a Correct Diagnosis

I am not here anymore.
Somewhere else is where I am.
A place so hard to find,
you cannot see me here
or visit me there
or wish me out of this anywhere.
If this is where I am supposed to be,
why can't I find me?

BETH ARRIVED for her doctor's appointment two hours late — and terrified. "I can't remember the day, or month, or sometimes even the year," she sputtered. "What's happening to me? Am I losing my mind? Am I crazy?"

Her physician, trying to offer reassurance, said, "You're seventy, Beth. What do you expect? You can't perform like a twenty-year-old anymore."

Like all of us, Beth wanted to perform as she always had, regardless of her age. A serious decline in mood, cognition, or functional behavior is *not* a normal part of aging; it indicates an underlying medical problem.

According to the National Alzheimer's Association, Alzheimer's disease has ten warning signs:

- Loss of memory
- Difficulty performing familiar tasks
- Problems with language
- Disorientation to time and place
- Poor or declining judgment
- Problems with abstract thinking
- Misplacing things
- Changes in mood and behavior
- Changes in personality
- Loss of initiative

An impairment in or loss of mental powers is called dementia, but dementia is a symptom, not a diagnosis. A finding of dementia cries out for more precise medical evaluation to rule out illnesses that may be not only treatable but curable. Larger metropolitan hospitals usually perform such an evaluation, called an Alzheimer's disease workup or AD workup, but residents of small communities may be able to find several different doctors who can collectively conduct the necessary tests. Call your nearest Alzheimer's Association chapter for specific information on where to find help in getting a diagnosis.

The evaluation includes a physical examination, psychological and neurological exams, and a complete medical history (including hospitalizations, serious illnesses, family members' illnesses and causes of death, and so forth), and a social history (education, military service, organizations joined, and so forth). Neurologists look for possible changes in the brain through magnetic resonance imaging (MRI) and possibly other scanning techniques. Other clinicians investigate medications used, nutrition, alcohol intake, metabolic disturbances, depression, and other possible causes of dementia.

Not only will the workup confirm Alzheimer's disease if it is present, but the exams should be able to identify whether the apparent problem has another cause.

Other conditions that can appear to be Alzheimer's disease include the following:

- Alcohol abuse
- Drug interactions
- Emotional problems/depression
- Endocrine imbalance
- Infection
- Metabolic disorder
- Poor nutrition or dehydration
- Trauma (emotional or physical)

Left untreated, many of these conditions can lead to irreparable physical or mental damage or even death. Unlike Alzheimer's, some of them can be cured.

Carrie joined an Alzheimer's support group and, at her first meeting, described how her family had "diagnosed" their mother, Therese. "It didn't take a medical degree," she told the other members. She and her brothers had not wanted to subject their mother to a lot of poking and prodding. "She's seventy-nine years old and the family doctor has known her for years," Carrie explained. "He told us that her forgetfulness and language problems are typical of Alzheimer's."

The other members tried to persuade Carrie to seek a more complete neurological evaluation. After three more meetings, Carrie gave in, if only "to prove to you all that Mother really does have Alzheimer's." She scheduled a visit with a memory-disorder clinic at a local teaching hospital, and with the help of a CAT (computerized axial tomography) scan, the doctors there discovered a small tumor growing in Therese's brain. She received the appropriate treatment and slowly returned to her old self, free of dementia and free of Alzheimer's.

Until recently, a diagnosis of Alzheimer's was quite difficult to prove; it could only be done definitively after death. The German neurologist Alois Alzheimer first identified the disease just about a century ago, in 1906, when he examined the brain of a deceased fifty-one-year-old woman whose "early-onset dementia" he had been following for many years. During the autopsy he discovered that nerve-cell fibers in her brain were entwined in what he called "neurofibrillary tangles." He named the areas of marked deterioration "plaques." Tangles and plaques remain the markers of Alzheimer's disease at autopsy. (We now know that plaques consist of a protein that goes awry, a malfunction that some scientists attribute to a genetic defect. As the plaques accumulate, brain function deteriorates.)

Some Early Tests for Alzheimer's

In recent years, doctors have become better able to identify Alzheimer's disease in living people. I do not give detailed or cutting-edge medical advice in this book — my expertise is in care partnering — but here are some tests that you may want to discuss with your physician.

- A lumbar puncture in the later stages of the disease that looks for amyloid and tau protein deposits, which are hallmarks of Alzheimer's
- An examination of tissue from the nasal passages
- A bone marrow test
- A commercial "sniff" test that can indicate certain types of dementia, which is readily available in drugstores
- A "Seven-Minute Screen" (contact your local Alzheimer's Association for details) that indicates whether further diagnostic tests are advisable
- A saliva test, given to people whose parents or siblings have developed Alzheimer's at an early age, that looks for genetic markers or hereditary factors.

As researchers try these tests on more patients, medical journals, the media, and the National Alzheimer's Association and its local chapters will alert the public and health care providers to the diagnostic value of each test. At present, too little is known about their efficacy for me to recommend any of them unequivocally.

Scientists have now determined that in people with Alzheimer's, nerve cells in the brain may start dying long before intellectual functioning changes noticeably, so the sooner a diagnosis is made and treatment begins, the better the chances are that the treatments will make a difference.

If you feel you are showing some early signs of the disease and you have a family history of Alzheimer's, consult with your physician to help you decide if you want to be tested. Evidence shows that if a parent, brother, or sister — first-degree relatives — develops Alzheimer's disease at an early age, you have a greater probability of developing the disease. If a family history of symptoms that we now recognize as Alzheimer's disease can be traced back for several generations, the incidence in future generations rises considerably. The genetic marker ApoE4 now helps detect familial Alzheimer's in families with a history of the disease.

More than a decade ago, my friend Charlie Pierce began wondering if he might develop Alzheimer's disease, since his father and siblings had had it. Charlie's book, *Hard to Forget*, about familial Alzheimer's, has given us all a more concrete and humane understanding of people like Charlie, still symptom free, who live each day knowing they may be the next one in the family to show signs of Alzheimer's.

A host of scientists are now using state-of-the-art technology to examine all potential causes of Alzheimer's, including genetic, viral, biochemical, and environmental problems, hoping to better understand the disease and find new treatments and, if possible, ways to halt or cure it. Genetic engineers and genomic researchers continue to delve into the recesses of the brain and the uncharted pathways of the body to find answers before people like Charlie have to deal, one more time, with familial Alzheimer's. This book cannot address all of the cutting-edge research that is being done, but certainly, if you have a family history of Alzheimer's, consult with your physician to determine the best course of action.

Products That May Alleviate Symptoms

A number of products — herbs, vitamins, and medicines — have been tested and found to provide some relief from certain early symptoms of Alzheimer's. None can be considered a cure, although they have shown some promise in reducing brain-cell damage. *These products should never be taken without consulting a physician, since any of them might be dangerous for a particular person.* The herbal products and vitamins include green-tea extract, selenium, grapeseed extract, and antioxidants such as vitamins A, C, and E. Researchers have not yet determined whether extract of *Ginkgo biloba* improves memory in people with Alzheimer's; studies show differing results. Also, because ginkgo is a blood thinner, it may cause more problems than improvements.

Some federally approved medications show varying amounts of success in reducing symptoms of Alzheimer's disease in some people and in keeping symptoms in others from getting worse. Each patient differs in the degree of responsiveness to the drugs and in the length of time they must be used before having any effect. Aricept, Exelon, and Reminyl work by increasing the amount of a bodily compound that is diminished in Alzheimer's patients, resulting in short-term memory loss. Anti-inflammatory medicines, including Celebrex and naproxen, may help by reducing swelling of the brain tissue associated with plaque formation. These drugs may slow the progression of the disease or protect people from exhibiting any symptoms. In clinical trials, Axura, or memantine, has shown some promise in slowing deterioration in the middle to late stage of Alzheimer's, though it has not yet been approved by the U.S. Food and Drug Administration.

Some compounds may even reduce one's chances of getting Alzheimer's. Certain researchers have shown that cholesterol-lowering drugs (statins) can block the toxic effects of cellular processes associated with Alzheimer's. Eating fish such as mackerel, sardines, and other cold-water fish whose oils contain omega-3 fatty acids can also promote brain health.

The medications and supplements mentioned above are generally most useful during the early and middle stages of Alzheimer's — a period that generally lasts between five and ten years.

Anyone who receives a positive diagnosis of Alzheimer's needs to deal with a host of social matters immediately. A man named Bill summed up this situation for me. "I need to get on with living," he told me. "There are so many things I want to do while I still can." Like most people, he had long dreamed of taking a trip to Europe with his wife, taking his grandchildren to Disney World. Now he wasn't going to wait any longer to put those plans into action. "Getting this news is not fun, and it does not make me happy, but it sure as hell beats getting run over by a car without being prepared. Now I can get on with living for whatever time is left. I have all this really great stuff in my head."

Every newly diagnosed Alzheimer's patient should learn that he or she is not simply "going crazy," that any changes in functioning are rooted in a physical disease. Certainly knowing that one has a neurological disorder is far better than silently worrying about a vague and menacing fear. Although it's completely normal to want to avoid the hard, bright line of a diagnosis of Alzheimer's, once the patient receives a competent, correct diagnosis, it is possible to take some concrete, positive steps that can significantly improve his quality of life.

Once the diagnosis is clear, the time is right for the care partner to tell the afflicted person, "No matter what happens, I will be here for you."

· 3 ·

What to Expect:
Making the First Decisions

*I wish there
were Cliff Notes
to help cheat my way
through this disease.*

GARY WAS a sixty-one-year-old high school math teacher who chose early retirement when his forgetfulness began to be an issue in class. Over the course of a year, although he had remained kind and caring, he had neglected to correct midterm exams, unknowingly missed a teachers' meeting, continually forgot where he parked his car in the staff parking lot, and had growing difficulties with a curriculum he had used successfully for nineteen years. At home a burnt teapot, a microwave explosion, and several small kitchen fires had forced him to exist on a diet of cold foods.

Some faculty members began to talk about how slovenly Gary had become. Some wondered if he had developed a drinking problem. Others thought he might be depressed. "Whatever it is," one colleague said, "he's just not the same Gary. And I feel as if I've failed as his close friend. He always says he's 'just getting old' and abruptly changes the subject. I know something more is wrong, but he just won't discuss it." Gary was encountering the early stage of Alzheimer's.

Sherry, too, was in the first stage of the disease but, unlike Gary, she had long been a domineering person. For five decades as a homemaker she had invested her energies in her three sons and her husband, Howard, and had felt in control of her life. Unfortunately, as the boys matured, married, and began raising families of their own, she had tried to stay in control by becoming more demanding, and her sons and their wives had begun to see her as a busybody much too involved in their affairs.

Then the family noted that getting along with Sherry had become even more challenging. If she made a mistake and someone corrected her, she would leave the room, banging the door behind her. When she repeated a story, as she often did, and the boys reminded her, she would raise her voice and tell them to "get out now." Then her daughters-in-law noticed a large purple bruise that covered most of Howard's lower arm. He explained that Sherry had hit him on the arm with a croquet mallet. He brought up other worries, too. "She won't stop driving," Howard said. "Every time she goes out in the car I feel sure she'll kill someone. But I can't stop her."

Sherry's domineering behavior did not diminish as her cognitive abilities began to decline. Quite the contrary: as she became aware of "losing control," she was far more likely to try to control those around her, and she did so by angry outbursts. She was essentially saying, in the only way she could, "I am still the boss and don't you forget it."

As was the case with Sherry and Gary, it is often a colleague, friend, family member, or outside helper who is the first person to notice changes in mood or behavior that suggest progressive dementia. The person experiencing the mood variations probably is aware of them but cannot face what they may mean. He hopes that the idiosyncrasies are temporary matters that can be explained away — "I need a good long vacation" — although he may begin to take stock and shift his priorities.

The Progression of Alzheimer's Disease

Clinicians typically refer to three stages of Alzheimer's disease — early, middle, and late. Each stage may be as brief as one year or as long as ten years, and there are wide variations from individual to individual. The first changes that Alzheimer's patients tend to go through are listed in the table below, followed by changes that occur in the later stages. Recognize that the intensity of a change — sometimes subtle, sometimes profound — varies widely from case to case. For good reason the constant refrain of care partners is "The most predictable part of Alzheimer's disease is the unpredictability."

Behavioral Change	Probable Stage
Not remembering appointments	Early
Not recognizing once familiar faces	
Losing track of time	
Not storing recent information or events	
Getting lost	
Having difficulty finding words	
Misplacing needed items	
Being unable to make decisions or choices	Middle Early
Finding it hard to concentrate	
Acting accusatory or paranoid	
Being unable to separate fact from fiction	
Being unable to translate thoughts into actions	
Misunderstanding what is being said	
Making mistakes in judgment	
Withdrawing, being frustrated and/or angry	Late Early
Losing ability to sequence tasks	
Speaking in rambling sentences	
Misusing familiar words	
Having difficulty writing	
Requiring supervision for "activities of daily living"*	
Showing impaired computing abilities	
Reacting less quickly	

Behavioral Change	Probable Stage
Losing fine motor skills (such as buttoning a shirt) Having more serious difficulties with ADL Not recognizing objects for what they are Being unable to understand written words Possibly displaying more sexual interests	Early Middle
Engaging in repetitive speech and action Having hallucinations and delusions Having problems with social appropriateness Experiencing altered visual perception Showing frequent changes of emotion Having minimal attention span Reacting catastrophically (overreacting, having outbursts) Needing assistance with all ADL Exhibiting frustration, anger, or withdrawal Walking with a shuffling gait	Middle Middle
Being incontinent Being mostly unintelligible Exhibiting a downward gaze Being unable to separate or recognize sounds	Late Middle
Losing all language Losing gross motor skills (sitting, walking) Having swallowing difficulties Needing total care	Late or Final

*Activities of daily living, or ADL, include bathing, dressing, grooming, eating, toileting.

After a diagnosis of Alzheimer's disease is made, the afflicted person (or her family or friends) should quickly start to look into some important matters concerning her care. Because many aspects of the Alzheimer's patient's daily care will not be performed at home, and because the patient may at some time need professional care, thoughtful financial planning from the start is important.

No matter how small the patient's resources are, a financial planner or elder-care attorney may provide compelling, unexpected reasons why someone else should manage the finances.

Keep in mind that not all nursing facilities will accept a patient who has no personal funds and who therefore must rely on Medicaid (state-provided medical assistance). The care partner needs to be sure that funds will be available when they are most needed — and that the question of who controls those funds has been decided. Addressing financial issues in depth is beyond the scope of this book (see Further Resources, page 212). At the first opportunity, contact a financial planner you can trust, and make the necessary arrangements.

The person with Alzheimer's should authorize someone trustworthy to make financial and medical decisions when she becomes unable to do so by a power of attorney or other appropriate documents. The patient might also create a living will, which may dispose of no-longer-needed assets and items while she is still alive. The Five Wishes Living Will (see Further Resources, page 225), which is valid under the laws of most states, also takes into consideration the person's emotional and spiritual needs. It provides specific instructions for the time of death, such as levels of comfort, life support, and other important factors. A health care proxy (which may be associated with either a power of attorney or a living will) allows the person to name someone she knows and trusts to make medical decisions. Of course, the legal needs of individuals vary, and each patient should consult a legal adviser on these matters.

At no time does an Alzheimer's patient feel more threatened than when facing the decision to stop driving — particularly when he either has not recognized or has denied that there's even a problem. When the habilitator confronts him, the subject generally becomes a battle — the patient will counter with verbal flare-ups and statements like "I've never had an accident before" or "I'm a much better driver than you are." Try not to argue with these kinds of statements. The issue now is not previous driving history, but what the future holds. The nature of the disease, which is hallmarked by problems with reflexes, judgment, way-finding, reaction time, decision-making, and other cognitive functions, will at some point make driving impossible.

Many people diagnosed with early-stage Alzheimer's decide to stop driving before they are in danger of getting lost or having an accident. But for many others, the issue is clouded by the overriding fear of losing independence and control over their life. The care partner must often find creative ways to keep the Alzheimer's patient from driving, perhaps by keeping the keys out of sight, getting into the driver's seat first, disabling the car by disconnecting the distributor cap, or by finding a trustworthy scapegoat such as a physician who will write a "prescription" to stop driving. If she has her own vehicle and the family has another car, take hers away as soon as possible — getting it out of sight will help dissipate her longings to drive. "It's at the garage" buys time; "It's having a tune-up" buys patience. These stratagems are all ways to deal with the problem until such time as the person no longer expresses a desire to drive — and this will happen.

Drivers Fifty and Older: Self-Rating Form*

This is a great quiz to help determine whether you should stop driving.

Instructions
For each of the following fifteen questions, check the symbol of the one answer that most applies to you.

Question	Always or Almost Always	Sometimes	Never or Almost Never
1. I signal and check to the rear when I change lanes.	◯	☐	☐
2. I wear a seatbelt.	◯	☐	☐
3. I try to stay informed about changes in driving and highway regulations.	◯	△	☐

Question	Always or Almost Always	Sometimes	Never or Almost Never
4. Intersections bother me because there is so much to watch from all directions.	○	△	○
5. I find it difficult to decide when to join traffic on a busy interstate highway.	□	△	○
6. I think I am slower than I used to be in reacting to dangerous driving situations.	□	□	○
7. When I am really upset, I show it in my driving.	□	□	○
8. My thoughts wander when I am driving.	□	△	○
9. Traffic situations make me angry.	□	△	○
10. I get regular eyesight checks to be sure my vision is sharp.	○	□	□
11. I check with my doctor or pharmacist about the effects of my medications on my driving ability. (*If you do not take any medication, skip this question.*)	○	□	□
12. I try to stay abreast of current information on health practices and habits.	○	△	□
13. My children, other family members, or friends are concerned about my driving ability.	□	△	○

Question	None	One or Two	Three or More
14. How many traffic tickets, warnings, or "discussions" with officers have you had in the past two years?	○	△	□

Question	None	One or Two	Three or More
15. How many accidents have you had during the past two years?	○	□	□

Self-Scoring
Count the number of check marks in the squares and record the total in the square below. Follow the same procedure for the triangles and circles.

□ △ ○ These are your check-mark totals. For score and interpretation, see the next section.

Step 1: In the square to the right, write the check-mark total recorded in the previous square.

□ × **5** = ___

Step 2: In the triangle to the right, write the check-mark total recorded in the triangle above.

△ × **3** = ___

Step 3: Multiply the number in the square by 5.

Step 4: Multiply the number in the triangle by 3.

Step 5: Add the results of Steps 3 and 4. **YOUR SCORE IS** ___

Interpretation of Your Score
The *lower* your score, the safer you are as a driver. The *higher* the score, the more dangerous you are to yourself and others.

Score	Meaning
0 to 15	GO! You are aware of what is important to safe driving and are practicing what you know.
16 to 34	CAUTION! You are engaging in some practices that need improvement to ensure safety.
35 and over	STOP! You are engaging in too many unsafe driving practices. You are a potential or actual hazard to yourself and others.

These scores are based on what drivers fifty-five years old and over have told the Foundation for Traffic Safety about their driving practices and habits. Your score is based on your answers to a limited number of important questions. A complete evaluation of your driving ability would require many more questions, along with medical, physical, and licensing examinations. Nevertheless, your answers and score give some indication of how well you are doing and how you can become a safer driver.

In general, a checked square for an item reflects an unsafe practice or situation that should be changed immediately. A checked triangle means a practice or situation that is unsafe or becoming unsafe. Checked circles are signs that you are doing what you should to be (and remain) a safe driver.

*This quiz is adapted from the quiz used by the Automobile Association of America (AAA)'s Foundation for Traffic Safety and is used with permission.

Formulating a Plan of Care

No matter what situation the care partner or family members find themselves in — caring for the person with Alzheimer's at home, in an assisted-living situation, or in a nursing home or similar facility — it is important to develop a plan of care. Care partners can use the plan to make sure that the patient's physical, social, emotional, and spiritual needs are being met *over a specific period of time.* Because the behaviors and needs of people with Alzheimer's change constantly as the disease and symptoms progress, the plan must be reviewed and updated on a regular basis — this is its primary purpose.

In the beginning, it may not be necessary to write out the plan of care — it can emerge from discussions with others involved in the caregiving process. If you do put the plan in writing, it could be as simple as "Continue with day care three times a week — no other changes."

Think of the plan of care as the routine you want the person with Alzheimer's to have. Initially, the routine should be close to whatever routine the person followed before the diagnosis. As the disease progresses, certain symptoms become apparent and certain behaviors become more problematic; for example, the patient may begin "sundowning" (becoming more aggressive in the evening). At this point you'll want to vary the routine to incorporate the change — by not inviting friends to visit during that time, for instance.

To develop a plan of care, consider the following needs:

- Physical: Is the person with Alzheimer's doing all right physically? Is she clean? Clothed? Eating regularly? Sleeping well? Having regular sexual intercourse, if desired?
- Social: Does the person with Alzheimer's have adequate social contacts? Does he seem withdrawn? Unhappy? Overly aggressive? Would modifying his social interactions positively change the behavior?
- Emotional: Is the person with Alzheimer's all right emotionally? Some of the questions here are the same as those concerning social needs; what is at stake here is whether the person's needs for love, intimacy, comfort, independence, easing of paranoid feelings, and so forth are being met.
- Spiritual: Does the person with Alzheimer's have adequate opportunities to fulfill spiritual needs? This aspect of the plan of care may be hard to quantify. Spiritual needs may range from attending religious services to feeding the birds: whatever spiritual sustenance maintained her before the disease began.

On a regular basis, assess the plan of care and modify it as necessary. For example, in January Corinne was taking care of her father, Rick. She kept him clean and fed (meeting his physical needs), regularly walked with him and some friends in a nearby park, took him to his favorite restaurant once a week (meeting his social and emotional needs), and allowed him time to putter around in his workshop/den (meeting his spiritual needs). In February, when Corinne assessed her plan of care, she noticed that her father had been acting more aggressive and more disoriented at the restaurant. She decided to go there only once every two weeks and substitute a take-out order at home for the second restaurant excursion. In March she realized that the two visits to the restaurant had become too difficult, so she removed them from her plan of care altogether.

The assessment of the plan of care will vary from care partner to care partner, and situation to situation. If the patient is being cared for at home, the habilitator should revisit the plan of care once a month. Assisted-living facilities and nursing homes generally use the plan of care as the basis for the patient's daily life, determining the patient's participation in recreational programs, menus, medications, and so forth. The usual policy is to review the plan of care once every three months.

For home care, the monthly assessment of the plan provides an ideal occasion to discuss the situation with others who may be helping out — the teen who comes once a week to take Grandfather on a walk in the park, for example, or the sister who arrives every Tuesday to watch Dad for a few hours. This once-a-month casual meeting can allow the care partner and helper to recommit to the process for the next month — "Would you like to come Tuesdays between three P.M. and six P.M. this month?" The helper can plan on this time to change the status, if necessary; and if the helper is used to this regular schedule of assessment, any changes of schedule will be easier for everyone.

The care partner has to continually assess what skills the patient has lost and what skills remain. For instance, you should check to see whether the oven has been left on, if burn marks have appeared on the bottom of the teapot, if the refrigerator contains spoiled food, and if the home is no longer as clean as it used to be. Deterioration in any of these instrumental aspects of daily life should not cause panic, but they do signal potential safety problems that should be considered seriously. Such findings may mark the time to ask others to help out or to bring in a professional support system. The chart showing the progression of Alzheimer's on pages 22–23 can be used as a checklist of sorts to determine the need for reassessment and evaluation of the patient's current abilities.

· 4 ·

Habilitation, the New Approach

Take away my license,
but don't steal my independence.
I will let you drive.
But let me tell you
where I want to go.

THE STAFF was busily opening draperies, letting the first beams of morning light into the rooms inhabited by the forty-five residents on floor two of the nursing center.

"I want to see my mother," Mary said softly to no one in particular as she shuffled from her room, holding on to the wall.

Claire, a young nurse's aide who happened to pass by at that moment, took Mary's hand. Then she said, sympathetically, "Mary, your mother has been dead a long time."

"Don't be so fresh," Mary said, pulling her hand away. "You don't know what you're talking about."

"Try to remember, Mary. You haven't seen your mother in years. She died when you were in your forties. You're eighty-seven now."

Mary shoved Claire out of her path. "My mother was right

here this morning. We had breakfast together like always. Now, get out of my way."

Gently, Claire took Mary's arm and began to guide her to the large-print calendar hanging in the nurses' station.

"No. I'm not going with you."

Claire tightened her grip. "I want to show you the date. Your mother died a long time ago."

Mary sputtered, "You — you — you — *hussy!*" Then, swinging her free arm, Mary caught the aide with a backhand slap to the face.

Claire called for help. Her colleagues responded and quickly subdued Mary, injecting her with an antipsychotic medication. For the rest of the morning, the staff kept Mary restrained to a chair in front of the nurses' station, where they could see her.

Until recently, this kind of scene occurred often in nursing homes where, in dealing with residents who might harm themselves or others, staff followed a protocol known euphemistically as "appropriate care." Claire's part of the dialogue with Mary followed a theory called "reality orientation." Staff members were taught to enforce a sense of the here and now. The idea was to make sure that all residents knew where they were, what food they had had for breakfast, the date, the day of the week, the year, and the name of the president of the United States.

"Your mother has been dead for years" is a prime example of reality orientation, although the person being addressed is far beyond being able to process the information. Sadly, the primary effect of forcing Mary to "face the truth" of her mother's long-ago death led to an escalation in her negative behavior. Her outburst was a way of defending herself against what she saw as a lie. Guided by emotion, her words failing, she reacted physically. In her internal reality, her mother was alive and they had enjoyed breakfast together earlier that morning.

Reality orientation is the antithesis of habilitation. Habilitation teaches care partners to place themselves in the patient's world, no matter where that world is. This teaching — live in the patient's world — is the fourth tenet of habilitation, as discussed in Chapter 1. The habilitative approach also acknowledges that reasoning with someone who has lost the power to reason only ensures confrontation.

Now imagine the same scene with staff members trained in the habilitation model of care.

When Mary expressed her wish to see her mother, the nursing aide said simply, "Tell me about her."

"She's a great cook," Mary said.

"What does she make that you especially like?"

"Oh, her pies are the best," Mary recalled. "I can never match 'em. Oh, dear, now I'm getting hungry."

Claire took Mary's hand and guided her toward the dining room. "Me too," she said. "You have a cup of coffee while I go get your friend Pat — we'll be right back."

Dignity intact, free from medical or chemical restraint, Mary sat back with her coffee and awaited her friend's arrival. Thoughts of her mother faded, replaced by the positive experience of Claire's smiling face and extended hand.

Following the tenets of habilitation, Claire made no attempt to "correct" Mary's sense of time and place or to reason with someone who no longer had that ability. At the same time, though, the aide validated Mary's emotional responses — her feeling of loneliness and her need for nurturing. Claire also bypassed a situation in which Mary could have felt a sense of failure. In taking this approach, the aide heeded the second, fourth, and fifth habilitation tenets: know that communication remains possible, live in the patient's world, and enrich the patient's life.

It is important to note as well that Mary required less time and fewer staff resources with the habilitation model — a compelling advantage in an era when the people who run nursing homes and other care facilities complain that there is never enough time or enough staff to practice new methods. Habilitation is by far the most effective approach for people in the early stages of the disease, when they are struggling to maintain their independence.

The habilitative method is significantly helpful when the patient's daily activities involve engagement with the rest of the world. Although such tasks as shopping, banking, doing the laundry, and driving will become increasingly more difficult as Alzheimer's progresses, by integrating the help of others and providing some simple cues, the care person can make daily tasks easier.

For example, one late afternoon Judy and Paul were preparing for visitors. The sun was shining in as Judy settled herself on the sofa across from the window while Paul made tea. The visitors arrived, and everyone sat down and began to talk, sipping tea and eating cookies.

Suddenly Judy rose and walked directly across the room to where one of the visitors was seated and shoved him squarely on the forehead, yelling, "Stop it! Stop it!"

Paul led her out of the room. The visitors excused themselves and graciously left the house, accepting Paul's apologies. Once, Paul would have seen Judy's behavior as "part of the disease" — but now, after several months of support group meetings, he knew how to look for what had triggered her outburst. When he returned to the living room, he sat where Judy had been seated on the sofa and immediately noticed that the sun shone directly in his eyes from the spot where the visitor had been sitting. Judy's way of ridding herself of the discomfort of the sun in her eyes was to try to beat it away. Paul's solution was to close the shade. By doing so, he successfully minimized both Judy's stress and his own.

As you'll see in later chapters, the patient may be able to live independently for longer and feel more in control if the care person modifies the environment in useful ways. For example, consider how you can help an afflicted person continue to do laundry, a task that can help make him feel like a helpful, important part of the housekeeping effort. Here are some suggestions:

- Keep laundry detergent in plain sight near the washing machine.
- Number the different boxes and bottles to be used; detergent, for example would be labeled #1, and softener would be #2.
- Write out a simple, clear list of steps for doing the laundry, and place the list near the washer and dryer.
- Mark the most frequently used washer and dryer settings with red nail polish or paint.
- Stick to a routine, doing the laundry on the same day each week and at the same time of day.

Consider how habilitation might have worked for Linda and her mother, Diane. "My daughter won't let me do the laundry anymore," Diane moaned at a patient support group meeting. "She says it makes more work for her when I do it. She claims I put whites in with colors, but I know I don't do that. She says I forget the detergent. Imagine that. 'Don't go near the wash while I'm out, Mama,' she says to me, as if I'm a child. I might as well put the TV on and sit like a lump all day if no one thinks I can do anything."

As Diane's ability to sequence the chore eroded, she probably was making the laundry chore harder for her daughter. But rather than emphasizing Diane's mistakes, the focus should be on what strengths she still had. Linda could give her mother the clean laundry and ask her to fold it — a repetitive task that Diane could still accomplish. Yes, she would take an hour longer than her daughter to finish the chore, but time is not the issue. Dignity is. Linda would praise Diane at the end and thank her for helping out. As a result both Linda and Diane would feel good.

Even for people with Alzheimer's disease, life is about doing, not just being. "What can I do — to help, to serve, to feel like a contributing part of family and community" is the silent plea of people with progressive dementia. Just receiving basic comforts and palliative care is not enough; these people need to feel useful to whatever extent is possible for them.

Focusing on What Remains

Family members often report to the doctor or nurse that the person with Alzheimer's disease cannot perform certain seemingly routine tasks long before the disease's normal progression suggests the need for hands-on assistance. In the parlance of health care professionals, this problem is called "excess disability." In an effort to keep the patient from attempting a task that might prove difficult, a well-meaning care partner may simply do the work for him. Although this might seem the best solution in the short term, it is likely to mean that the patient will soon not be able to perform the task at all.

Consider how habilitative principles could have helped Peter. His disease had led him into a world in which some of the simplest activities of daily living had become sources of frustration. In response, he strove even harder to maintain his independence, resisting the efforts of his family members who, he thought, were determined to infantilize him.

One morning Peter woke up early, as usual, and went into the bathroom before anyone else arose. This was his way of trying to take care of himself on his own. Once in the bathroom, he stood in front of the sink, wondering what to do next. He vaguely recognized where he was, yet he wasn't sure why he was there. After a while his pajama pants felt wet and warm.

Next he examined the many objects in front of him. He was

unsure which ones were used for what purposes. Aha. "Tooth stuff," he muttered as he picked up and squeezed a red and white tube. He cautiously smeared on his teeth the green paste coming out of the tube.

A few minutes later, Peter became thoroughly annoyed at the wetness and the cold feeling of his pajama pants. He tried to slide the pants off, but a drawstring fastened them tightly at the waist. He sat down on the edge of the tub and began to tug harder and harder until the cloth tore apart. He smiled with satisfaction as the cotton began to shred into long strips suspended from his waist.

Suddenly his wife, Abby, burst through the bathroom door. Horrified, she shouted, "Look what you've done. You've ruined a perfectly good pair of pajamas. And you have toothpaste all over your face. What am I going to do with you?"

She started to wash and dress him, calling for her daughter to come in and help, doing just what Peter most feared — treating him like a baby. If Peter could have articulated his feelings, I think he would have said, "I am still here. I am not gone. I'd rather try and fail than have you do these things for me. Please give me the chance to do one little thing for myself, and if I end up with my BVDs on my head, so what? Imagine how good I feel doing things myself. Please focus on how I feel and not on how I look."

Using the principles of habilitation, Abby could have helped Peter retain more independence in his personal habits. If he had had elastic-waist pajama bottoms, he could easily have removed them himself when the wetness made him uncomfortable. Abby could have placed toothpaste on his toothbrush, laid the brush on the sink top, and put the paste out of sight. She could have re-moved the other bathroom items, putting his brush, comb, shav-ing cream, and safety razor (which isn't dangerous if he has always used one) on the vanity.

While Peter was grooming, his daughter could have laid out

his day's clothes, sequencing the items by placing the first article of clothing he would put on — his briefs — on top, followed by his undershirt, trousers, and socks — in the order Peter had always put them on. When he had completed his basic dressing routine, his daughter could have held up two appropriate shirts and asked, "Which would you like to wear today, Dad?" assuring that her father still felt in control and able to make personal choices.

In this scenario, everyone would have won: completing the task would have preserved Peter's vital self-esteem, and he could have conducted his toileting and dressing without Abby's using negative words or losing her temper. The objective of habilitation is to find each patient's optimal ability to function independently. Clinicians gauge how well a person can get along in a home setting according to how well she can perform specific activities of daily living. (For detailed suggestions and help with activities of daily living, see Chapter 8.)

Sometimes it is difficult to figure out how much independence the Alzheimer's person can use, as Michaela described at a care-partner support group. Her husband, Laurence, had repeatedly said he wanted to use their snow blower to clear the driveway of the heavy snow that had fallen. She finally decided to let him do this, so she started the machine for him and gave him initial instructions.

Back indoors, she realized that the blower's hum seemed rather distant. Looking out the window, she noticed six feet of snow piled in front of their neighbor's garage doors, where Laurence was blowing the snow from the driveway. Michaela still wanted her husband to succeed at the task, so when he begged for a second chance, she gave him simple, clear instructions on how to blow the snow from their own driveway onto the lawn. But some minutes later she again found him at their neighbor's, this time blowing all the snow from the lawn onto the driveway, which had been professionally plowed earlier that morning.

Once again Michaela walked over to the neighbor's yard; gently taking hold of the snow blower handle, she shut off the engine. "Laurence," she said, "the engine seems to be overheating. Let's give the machine a rest." As she took his hand, she said, "I need a cup of coffee. How about you? Want some chocolate cake?" Together they began trudging home through the snow, leaving the blower and the comical scene for her teenage son to remedy.

Every care partner must find a balance between allowing the person with Alzheimer's enough independence to have opportunities to succeed, but not so much as to cause new failures. Formulating and consistently revising a workable plan of care will help the habilitator assess the person's abilities.

The care partner should also look for repetitive tasks that the patient can do successfully. Tasks that do not require a great deal of supervision allow the person with Alzheimer's to still feel independent and useful, with minimum assistance from others. Repetitive tasks, such as rolling dough for pie crust or raking autumn leaves, are often the best choice to compensate for cognitive losses such as attention span and sequencing. Any activity that offers the patient a chance to feel useful and successful — dusting, sandpapering, vacuuming, weeding, shoe polishing, or sorting objects — can be rewarding activities if the care partner makes them so.

One evening I entered my kitchen after dinner to find my husband standing at the sink with my brand-new Teflon-coated frying pan in one hand and a wire scrubber in the other. Teflon cookware was fairly novel in the early 1970s, and I had saved to purchase this one. My heart sank when I saw him. But he was smiling as he began the task of getting the Teflon off the pan — scrubbing and scrubbing, smiling and smiling. The task took him about two hours to complete. By the time he left the kitchen, proudly holding the frying pan in the air and proclaiming victory over Teflon, I had bathed a toddler, looked over homework assignments, ironed shirts for the next school day, and finished a host of other chores. I hugged him and told him it was the best darn job I had ever seen. The kids joined me in applause.

The next morning he was still smiling, though I don't think he remembered what had made him so happy. But that wasn't important. Praise and thanks go a long way in combating injured self-esteem and feelings of helplessness.

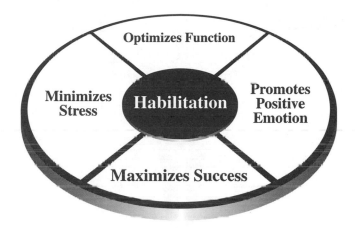

The habilitative model produces critically important results.

Domains

As the care partner fosters independence and self-respect, another aspect of habilitation to consider is what my friend and colleague Dr. Paul Raia calls "domains." While the five tenets are the *tools* that care partners will use to make the Alzheimer's patient function in the best way possible, the six domains discussed on the following pages are the *locations* — either physical or mental — in which the tenets can be implemented.

The Six Domains

Physical issues, such as grooming and dressing, and the patient's emotional styles are the foundation blocks of a meaningful habilitation program, along with functional support, which includes elements of the environment such as paint, lighting, and colors. With those three "bricks" in place, the care partner can concentrate on the patient's sense of the world and his interactions with others. When the bricks are balanced, the patient can communicate meaningfully with others even without using words. But if one brick is removed, the others will fall down as well.

1. The Physical Domain

As the disease progresses, surroundings that were once a familiar aspect of the patient's daily existence become less familiar, leaving him with feelings of apprehension and confusion. At this point, he is likely to act out frequently, expressing fear or dismay through an outburst of agitation or aggression.

Since these acts are the patient's way of seeking self-protection, the care partner can try to reduce his anxiety by recognizing that he is probably having growing problems with visual perception (the ability to see contrasts, colors, depth, and motion), cognition (intellectual functioning), and orientation (familiarization to people, places, or time).

Painting a bathroom wall a deep or bright color can draw the patient's attention to the contrasting white toilet, for instance. Enhancing personal areas with memorabilia, eliminating clutter, illuminating task areas, and doing away with sources of shadows can also help. Such changes give patients the greatest chance of being able to function at their highest level for a longer time. Chapter 6 discusses these ideas in more detail.

2. The Functional Domain

The routines that the person followed before she was afflicted by Alzheimer's should be the foundation for keeping her active in her own care and thus relatively independent for as long as possible.

The care partner can offer simple prompts to foster the patient's remaining skills in activities of daily living, which include bathing, dressing, eating, toileting, and sleeping. Place the toothpaste on her toothbrush before she goes into the bathroom for morning grooming. Lay out her clothes in the order that she will put them on. Schedule her shower at the time when she is most relaxed, alert, and cooperative (usually when she wakes up in the morning, before the day's challenges begin). At the dining table, the habilitator should eliminate meaningless utensils and many condiments, because several choices may prove to be overstimulating. And if the patient fails at complicated tasks, assist her with a simpler version of the chore. For instance, if planting the vegetable garden becomes overwhelming, perhaps she can help decide what vegetables to plant.

3. The Social Domain

Almost all of us have an innate desire to be social. We perform better, laugh more, and feel more emotionally secure when we feel the closeness of other people and, perhaps, pets. This desire for closeness does not disappear when someone develops Alzheimer's disease. Many health care professionals in this field report that even patients who are said by their families to be quite unsocial or who have lived for decades without close friends, as well as those who live reclusively because of their illness, have enjoyed relationships with new friends and old family members as the disease progresses. With the loss of inhibition and control, perhaps these patients can now enjoy the company of others, feeling more grounded and safe when people are around.

People with progressive dementias who spend much of their time doing nothing show many more signs of anxiety, depression, and paranoia than their counterparts who are occupied in daily chores and activities. Too much leisure time adds to the patient's feeling of being devalued as a noncontributing family or community member. Everyone, including people with Alzheimer's, needs opportunities to feel successful.

To prevent social problems from building, care partners should constantly include patients in conversation and have friends in to visit one on one. Reminiscing, enjoying music, engaging with children or pets, pursuing hobbies, or participating in religious events can provide feelings of enrichment and accomplishment. Such responses help the patient remain oriented and engaged, maximizing his or her strengths while minimizing isolation.

4. The Communication Domain

Our ability to communicate with language sets us apart from other animals. The loss of language, therefore, can feel dehumanizing. But the habilitation model of care provides a profound opportunity for communication as a way to elicit positive emotions. The habilitator's tone of voice, gestures, and facial expressions can help counteract the patient's failing language patterns. The care partner can also communicate with pictures rather than words. The method chosen should be appropriate to the individual, and it must change as his communication abilities alter. For instance, a patient who has just begun to need some assistance with word finding may find it demeaning to have words replaced with pictures. In a more advanced stage, however, looking at pictures of infants, for example, may elicit far more delight than trying to have a conversation about babies.

The overall goal is maintaining the emotion of personal value, and the less frustration the patient experiences from verbal errors, the longer he will continue to interact with others. A care partner will not be able to change the imperfect language of a person with Alzheimer's, but the helper can do much to modify his or her reaction to this ongoing loss.

5. The Sensory Domain

Researchers have long identified the senses as an area of particular interest. This domain involves both receiving the sensory signals — sights, sounds, odors, tastes, and textures — and processing these signals in the brain. Alzheimer's disease may scramble the processing of these signals to the point that the patient is unable to share information about what she is seeing, smelling, hearing, tasting, or touching. Yet sensory signals still enter the brain, and they may affect the person on a deep, emotional level, for good or ill.

For example, smell is the oldest and most powerful of our senses, and smells can be used to calm a patient. Once, after I visited one of my grandsons, my daughter dropped me off at the airport. As she drove back to their house, my daughter suggested to her teary six-year-old that they stop and buy a pizza. "No way," he replied. "I don't want anything in this car to take away the smell of Mummum." The fragrance of my bath powder in the car had evoked and sustained a pleasant memory for him. In the same way, many good Alzheimer's programs now use aromatherapy to help evoke pleasant memories.

As for hearing, at some point in the progress of the disease, the person will have difficulty separating one sound from another. Then the care partner needs to minimize distracting or overstimulating noises that may unnerve him. The same effort to minimize and simplify will help those in whom the disease has altered the ability to interpret color, shape, contrast, and motion. For instance, the person may perceive shadows and lights as threatening. If his tactile senses are affected, he may not be able to identify items in his pockets. Someone whose taste buds have changed may enjoy his food more if it is enhanced with herbs and spices.

As the disease progresses, perceptions become ever more problematic until, finally, messages from all of the senses become tangled.

6. The Emotional Domain

As I've suggested, problems in the other domains can lead to emotional problems if a care partner does not use the habilitative approach. In my experience, it is habilitators' unrealistic expectations that most often trigger frustration, verbal agitation, and physical aggression. Most behavioral changes in a person with progressive dementia are rooted in the frustration of being unable to master an emotional and physical environment that feels like foreign territory.

An afflicted person may ask her lifelong spouse, "Who are you?" Or say, "I don't belong here," gesturing to the kitchen of the house where she's lived for forty-seven years. The statement may be cognitively absurd, but the underlying emotion — in these cases, fear — is real. Such statements are both clues to the person's emotional state and warnings that a behavioral change, driven by apprehension, is about to occur.

The habilitation approach accepts that a care partner can influence behavior only indirectly, by changing the patient's environment and by adjusting his or her own attitudes. Trying to use rewards to reinforce positive behavior makes no sense after the point when patients can no longer understand the link between a behavior and a positive reinforcement.

For example, if Travis continually tries to open the door and get out of a moving vehicle, the answer is not to offer his favorite strawberry milkshake if he sits still for the duration of the ride. He no longer sees the connection between his behavior and the reward or lack of reward. The appropriate way to control this problem is to stop taking Travis for rides in the car for a while, until this particular behavior subsides. As for the milkshake — give it to him anyway.

Families and professionals must be aware of the ongoing need to reassess the patient's domains and to modify the care partner's actions and reactions. With education, practice, patience, and support, care partners can learn how to reach patients through their remaining capacity to feel and exhibit emotions.

5

Seeing the World from
the Patient's Perspective

I've danced,
I've sung,
I've given birth,
I've laughed,
I've succeeded.
Why is everyone
so sad?

AT AN EARLY-STAGE Alzheimer's group meeting, Jim described how people began to speak more loudly to him after they learned of his diagnosis. "One jerk even said to my wife, 'Ask him if he wants coffee.' I screamed back at him, 'Yes, I do — with sugar!' You should have seen the look on the guy's face." Jim chuckled. The rest of the group nodded with recognition. They had all experienced similar reactions.

To the patient, a diagnosis of progressive dementia means the recognition of a disease that is already active and that will, presumably, continue for a relatively long time. But too often, outsiders think they should start treating the person differently, without recognizing his existing abilities. Or they may worry that if they speak to him about the disease, they are being too personal. But speaking with and listening to the patient — allowing him to talk openly about feelings and abilities — helps significantly. In 1996, researcher Mary Mittelman, a professor of psychology at New York University Medical Center, published an article in the *Journal of the American Medical Association*, about the crucial importance of families and patients speaking and listening to one another about the diagnosis and the disease.

Listening is the best way for the care partner to seal a positive pact with the afflicted person. The language that the patient uses is of little importance. What matters is that someone is listening with heart and soul, unconditionally and without interruption. Listening tells the patient "I value you" louder and clearer than almost anything else. Listening also helps the care partner understand how the patient is reacting to this disease and to the way people treat her. This has an even greater impact since most people, including health care professionals, generally do not include patients in conversation. But people with Alzheimer's resent being seen as deaf and dumb. Many of them will talk much less than they did before the diagnosis, and some will stop talking completely, fearful that they will make mistakes.

In talking to a person with Alzheimer's, the goal is to stimulate conversation and win trust on a personal level before expecting her to open up. The particular subject isn't important; I often talk about movies I've seen or parties I've been to. Weddings are a favorite topic with women; ball games rate high with many men. Maintain eye contact to assure the patient that you truly are listening. Be aware of the expression your face is conveying. Every chance you have to nod or pat the patient's arm in affirmation will encourage confidence, and that will help the Alzheimer's person to speak out, even if language is a challenge.

Whenever other people are present, show them how to include the patient, even the most profoundly speech-deprived, by addressing him directly, referring to him, and incorporating him into the general laughter and body language. A wink is a great way to convey a sense of inclusion. The person with Alzheimer's disease — like anyone with memory loss — may soon forget what you say, but he will never forget how you made him feel.

Talking about the Disease

People with Alzheimer's will let their friends and loved ones know they want or need to talk about the disease. The dilemma is that the friend or family member may not be ready, or prepared, to talk about what is happening and may either deny that the person has the disease or just brush off the attempt to talk about it.

In an early-stage patient support group meeting, Rachel commented, "I long to have someone take my hand and say, 'This must be awful for you.' Instead, my daughter looks at me with tears in her eyes and goes into another room. When I ask my husband if I'm losing my mind, he says, 'We're all getting old' and that's the end of that. I know what's happening. Why won't my family talk about it?" Rachel went on to describe how, after her younger sister was diagnosed with cancer, the whole family rallied and helped her make plans. The contrast makes it all the more difficult for Rachel to comprehend the silence surrounding Alzheimer's.

If patients want to discuss the disease, most often they ask such questions as "Am I losing my mind?" "Am I going crazy?" "What's wrong with me?" Or their desire to talk may take the form of statements such as "I feel like I'm becoming senile," "I'm no good anymore," "I can't seem to think straight," or "I'm so forgetful these days."

No matter what form the comment takes, these personal assertions often have a single meaning: *Tell me why this is happening. Help me understand.* As soon as the person with Alzheimer's broaches the subject, say something like "The brain disease makes you feel that way. Let's talk about it." Talking about the disease helps relieve the patient's anxiety and can often deepen the relationship with the care partner.

A patient may try to broach the subject with her physician — and if the physician is skilled in communicating, that may be a good idea. The physician certainly can discuss the physical, mental, and emotional ramifications of Alzheimer's and may be able to offer intelligent, thoughtful comments and advice when others who are close to the patient feel tongue-tied and ill equipped to discuss these issues.

Since memory loss produces great anxiety, a normal coping mechanism is to try to hide the problem or deny that it is occurring frequently. One time Richard poignantly described how fearful he felt almost every moment as he declined. "Suddenly I'm having trouble remembering my neighbors, although I've lived beside them for thirty-six years. I glance over the evening paper at my wife and fight to recall her name. Still, there are times when I feel like my old self, ready to teach another chemistry class, ready to watch a Packers game, ready to win a hand of bridge. At those moments I think nothing is wrong, maybe I was just overtired. Sometimes things are losing meaning as I breathe. I wish I could tell the people around me how I'm feeling when these 'brain attacks' happen. I'm afraid I'll lose my job or won't be invited to play bridge anymore or will just be treated differently."

When attacks of memory loss increase to the point that they must be acknowledged, a patient's fear grows. At this point, a thoughtful care partner can make all the difference. I was impressed with the way Ernie's daughter, Stephanie, dealt with her father's memory problems without perturbing him.

Ernie was heading to the dining table for lunch when he saw a cardinal perched on the bird feeder outside the family-room window. "Wow, will you look at that!" he said. He followed the bird's flight from the feeder to the cherry tree and then to the neighbor's roof. When the cardinal was out of sight, he returned to his chair in the den, picked up the morning paper, and perused the front page. His soup grew cold on the dining room table.

Stephanie recognized Ernie's ability to focus on only one thing at a time. She reheated the soup, then appeared at his side and used verbal prompting to get him to eat the soup. "Come on, Dad, let's have lunch together." She prompted him without using any chiding or negativity. And calmly saying the word "lunch" was enough to trigger the memory of what he had been about to do before the cardinal captured his attention.

"Oh," he said sheepishly, "I was supposed to do that a while ago, wasn't I?"

Don't Worry about Rejection

Family members, friends, coworkers, and acquaintances are often put off by what appears to be the impaired person's lack of interest in them or downright rejection. Why wouldn't they be offended? After all, someone they have known for years seems now to be snubbing them, averting his eyes when they meet by chance, acting downright bizarre. At other moments, this strange person becomes once again the husband or friend or neighbor he has always been.

The more we understand that his behavior is a result of a disease process and not an intentional desire to be aloof, the more we can help the person who is losing his memory or his ability to focus. At the same time we can be relieved of wondering what we might have done to cause the rejection.

If the person with Alzheimer's has had an outburst when friends are visiting or in the company of others, don't remind her of the incident. Consider only what can be done to keep it from happening again. An outburst may be a direct response to her realization that she no longer fits in. Although she may not know exactly what to do, she may be very much aware of her loss of control. Becoming remote or seeming indifferent is a way of dealing with uncertainty about how to act.

When visiting someone else's home, even a familiar one, the Alzheimer's patient may have hallucinations (seeing or hearing something imaginary), delusions (believing something that is invalid — for example, "I hear people talking about me"), or even paranoid reactions (blaming others for something he himself has done or something he cannot make sense of — for example, "You're stealing all my money!" or "Where did you hide my keys?"). Explaining or trying to clarify what is happening will not help and may make the situation worse by increasing the person's anxiety.

A thoughtful habilitator can calm the anxiety, however, by addressing feelings of fear or sadness directly and by altering the environment in some way; emotion or the environment may be the cause of the hallucination, delusion, or paranoia. Remember that the altered state of perception is real to the patient — don't try to suggest otherwise.

One day Ginny told our care partner support group that her mother Rosalie had called her six times one morning. "Where are you?" Rosalie demanded. "Don't you understand? Someone is robbing me! I want you to do something about it *now.*"

"Mom, this is the sixth time you've called. If you'd stop calling long enough for me to get dressed and come over, I'll be right there."

"More things will probably be missing by then!" Rosalie shouted as she hung up.

Take a deep breath, Ginny told herself. *Poor Mom really believes that someone is stealing from her. I must not let my feelings get in the way of helping her through this. Denying that it is happening or reasoning with her sure hasn't helped in the past . . . in fact, it seems to make it worse. I wish I hadn't been so short with her on the telephone.*

Rosalie's front door was unlocked, so Ginny walked in.

"Oh, you scared me!" Rosalie said, starting in surprise. "How did you get in?"

"I walked in. The door was unlocked."

"It certainly was not! It was the burglars — they left it open. They've taken some silver and crystal and money and Lord only knows what else. This is the third time I've been robbed, and the police won't do a thing. What are you going to do, Ginny?"

Ginny knew Rosalie had forgotten that in previous incidents the police had conducted a brief search and found the "missing" objects, which had simply been misplaced. This time Ginny dutifully sat with her mother over a cup of tea and made a list of all the missing objects. Some of them she could see in the china closet, but she wrote them down anyway. Slowly the conversation turned to life in the city today and how it had changed over the years. Rosalie expressed some of her fears of living alone and Ginny again suggested door alarms so she would know if someone was trying to come in. This time Rosalie agreed, and Ginny returned later with the alarms.

Moving to a safer place with people her own age was beginning to sound like a better idea to Rosalie than it had the month before. Meanwhile her feelings had been validated, and Ginny felt one step closer to establishing a more appropriate environment for her mother. Rosalie's issues are typical among patients moving down the road of Alzheimer's disease.

Lights along the Way

Some people with Alzheimer's, fortunately, have jumped at the opportunity to give helpful suggestions for others on the same journey. Sometimes, they counsel, you may stumble, sometimes you will succeed, sometimes you will dance, and you will always need validation.

Over the past fifteen years, along with my colleagues Paul Raia, Elaine Silverio, and Lois Pecora, I have asked early-stage support groups about living with Alzheimer's. The insights the groups have offered have taught us a great deal. Following are some comments by people in these groups.

- I don't know how to act — I've never been here before.
- I cannot function when there is noise — even the sound of my own breathing scares me at times.
- I am waiting for the next shoe to fall.
- Not only is my brain getting smaller, but so is my world.
- Don't "test" me with questions — that does not make me better, it makes me sadder.
- I think my neighbors fear that I'm a madwoman.
- I am still here — parts of me are missing, but parts of me are still damn good.
- I never taught my children how to hear my pain. I was too busy telling them to listen.

These group members were asked what helps the person with Alzheimer's disease to function at the most optimal level, and what suggestions they would have to help others in their situation live more positively. They had the following tips:

- Share your diagnosis with friends and family. As Jake told us, "It is far better to have them walk with you through the disease than to have them run away from you because they think you are losing your mind or have had too many martinis at lunch."
- Cherish each moment. Don't waste a lot of time looking ahead or back. This minute is good only if you make it so, and a lot of little minutes add up to a full day.
- Know that some days or hours will be better than others. Even if today was not such a good day, tomorrow still can be.
- Find humor whenever possible, especially if it means laughing at yourself.
- A peaceful environment is much easier to function in, so keep sounds, like TV, to a low level.

- Tell those you love that you can do almost anything if the steps are easy.
- Have patience with your loved ones; they are learning, too.
- A pocket-size notebook may help you remember appointments or events. Keep this notebook with you at all times and write down everything that occurs during the day. Review your notes at night, highlighting facts that seem significant.
- Buy large-face clocks with black numbers on a white background or vice versa, to aid failing perception.
- Tell storekeepers about your memory problems. Chad carries a card that simply states "I have memory difficulties. Please be patient." He hands the card to wait staff and salespeople. "Most of the time," he says, "I try to revisit familiar places where they already know my condition."
- Increase your support circle by reconnecting with old acquaintances and family members. Long-term memory remains intact for a long time; old buddies can reinforce these memories and share tales of days gone by.
- A "one-day-at-a-time" calendar can help you focus on today and not let the bigger picture overwhelm you.
- Take advantage of every opportunity to feel uplifted. You know the adage about "taking time to smell the flowers." Well, don't forget to feed the neighborhood strays and examine snowflakes and consider the vast difference between an oak leaf and a mountain ash leaf. Steve says he never realized how many kittens came to visit his yard until he had Alzheimer's. "Now I feed every one of them, and I've named them all. I never quite recall their names from one day to the next, but they don't seem to care."
- Register with the Alzheimer's Association Safe Return Program (see Further Resources, page 217), even if you feel certain you will never get lost. This program helps find people

with memory impairment and provides a central structure for monitoring the search for a missing person. Communication with the family awaiting the return of loved one is an integral part of this program.

• A support group for patients is the perfect place for sharing your feelings and concerns. "I feel that I am not alone," says group member Ruth. "No one else ever asks me how I feel. In fact, no one ever seems to think that I do feel, and I feel deeply. My family is crying all the time about losing me — well, so am I."

We need to hear the patient when she asks us to listen. We must support her failing words. Instead of abandoning previous relationships, we need to expand them. We must be innovative, courageous, and flexible and realize that the patient is courageous, too.

We must know, deep in our gut, that the time when the afflicted person is the least lovable is probably the time when he needs love the most. This journey has no guideposts to help us along the way. But we can use our new perception to take slow steps together into this land of altered communication forms. We always need to be mindful that outside appearances give no real clue to what remains within.

PART TWO

The Five Tenets of Habilitation

■   ■   ■

6

Tenet #1: Make the Physical Environment Work

Sometimes, something is familiar to me.
Most times there is no recognition
of the fabric of my life.
Only frayed remnants of who I once was.

THE NEXT FIVE CHAPTERS discuss the five tenets of habilitation in detail and in the order that will allow a habilitator to
make use of them most easily. To work properly, however, the
tenets must be applied all together; the difficult part is often
learning how to apply them in a particular situation.

This chapter focuses on the physical world around the person
with Alzheimer's and gives specific suggestions for altering the environment to improve the quality of life for both patient and care
partner. To begin with, pay close attention to what the memory-
impaired person sees, hears, smells, and touches in a world that is
becoming increasingly less familiar. These clues will help you
adapt the environment to maintain a certain level of self-care,
create chances for feeling successful, and minimize distress.

Although none of us lives in the world that the Alzheimer's

patient now inhabits, we can try to understand how the disease may be affecting him. Imagine these difficult experiences:

- Looking at a staircase and seeing a wall.
- Gazing into a mirror to find what seems to be someone else staring back at you.
- Having someone tell you to sit down when you cannot find a chair.
- Hearing many sounds — television, voices, traffic — that others don't hear.
- Feeling keys in your pocket but not knowing what they are.
- Smelling the odor of mothballs in your grandmother's attic — but where is the attic and where is Granny?

Next, consider the feeling of having many senses bombarded at once and having ever greater difficulty separating today from yesterday. Doesn't it feel frustrating and scary? Remember these emotions whenever you interact with the patient. Even in the earliest stage of the disease, she may have some of these feelings. Try to see, feel, hear, taste, and touch as she is — and always remember that no matter how well she is performing, the disease is affecting her perspective, so it is different from your perception.

Next consider how the person's surroundings may affect the changes in perception. You can and should alter the environment so that it helps prevent problems for the patient. The overarching idea is to make the surroundings as simple as possible.

Lighting

Start by thinking through how lighting can help control behavior, increase safety, and offer comfort and a feeling of security to the patient. The goal of lighting is to mimic daylight, which is the most comfortable kind of light for patients. Many distributors now offer bulbs under such names as "day glow," "vita lite," or "pink light." You can also make a fluorescent ceiling fixture feel more like natural light by replacing the cover with a parabolic grid, which resembles rows of two-inch plastic cubes. The grid diffuses light and eliminates shadows. Focused-task lamps should be used only on a desk or a table where the patient works. Having a number of lamps on creates too many shadows, which an Alzheimer's patient may misinterpret or find threatening.

It may seem impractical to leave lights on at night, but accidental toileting problems are not practical either. Nighttime incontinence may just be the result of not being able to find the bathroom quickly enough. At most hardware stores you can purchase a roll of sticky-backed reflector tape, which you can run from bedside to bathroom to mark this most important path, illuminating it with several nightlights. Even better, 3M produces a reflector tape that needs little or no light; it is pricey but worth the cost.

Install dimmer switches throughout the house and turn up the lights as the sun starts to go down to help the patient who may become influenced by "sundown syndrome." Often a patient's aberrant behavior begins to surface at that time of day and may continue for several hours. "Sundowning" generally occurs between three o'clock in the afternoon and eight in the evening, depending on the season.

As part of the effort to simplify the environment as much as possible, try to replace floor lamps with lighting that is attached to the wall. That will help make the house as clutter-free as possible.

Color Schemes

You can also help an Alzheimer's patient by choosing indoor and outdoor color schemes carefully. Researcher Dr. Alice Cronin-Golomb, in the psychology department at Boston University, has found that the disease affects patients' reactions to colors. Sandra Harris, who specializes in interior design for Alzheimer's patients, has found that using unique colors for different areas and spaces can help keep the patient oriented in her home and can enable her to travel from one room to another without getting lost. Flat rather than high-gloss paint on walls helps eliminate both glare and shadows.

Try to find wall colors that contrast with the functional objects in a room. For instance, if the furniture in a room is light-colored wood, you may want to paint the walls deep aqua or a warm peach; if the room has dark, varnished wood furniture, then light-colored walls will provide a good contrast. Bright colors can help balance failing perception of depth and contrast. You may be able to help a patient's orientation by putting colorful cushions on dining chairs, choosing frames in primary colors for her favorite photos, and placing lively place mats under table lamps. The use of colors for definition and contrast will allow the patient to continue using household objects, such as cooking utensils, hobby materials, and small pieces of furniture, for much longer.

Paint the wall behind the toilet a darker, contrasting color so it's easy to spot from the bathroom doorway. If sofas and chairs blend with the background, use colorful throws or afghans to draw attention to where the patient should sit — his altered perception may make it difficult to decide.

Color can be used not only to highlight utilitarian items but also to camouflage objects to avoid. To keep a patient out of harm's way, you can place a black mat inside the front door to suggest a dark chasm that can't be crossed. Many fine long-term-care facilities specializing in the care of Alzheimer's patients have found this to be a great way to keep their residents from wandering off. Staff members report that the most positive aspect of using black mats is not having to issue negative commands. When the Alzheimer's resident sees the "hole," he simply turns back in the other direction.

Along the same lines, painting or wallpapering entry doors to match the surrounding walls makes them harder to see. Place functioning locks, and even doorknobs, up high or down low on doors, leaving the useless locks and knobs in place; the person will often believe that the nonfunctioning lock or knob is broken or stuck and will not see (or look for) the newly installed hardware.

If the patient's bedroom is kept simple, with only a splash of color on the bed to draw her attention, she will tend to use the room only for sleeping at night and dressing rather than for napping during the day.

Consider the following scenario:

Where's my underwear, Wanda?" Burt hollered.

"On the bed, where I always put it. Look on the bed."

Burt tore the bed apart. "It's not here! Where is it? I'm stark naked."

Wanda came into the room. "Look, it's right where I put it. Here on the pillow."

Wanda had made the mistake of placing the white briefs on a white pillow, making it very difficult for Burt to see them. Had she laid Burt's white briefs on top of the navy bedspread, he would easily have spotted his underwear on the contrasting visual field.

By and large, stick to a palette of solid, strong, simple colors. If you are able to visit a paint store and look at paint sample cards, the middle section, working toward the darker end, will include the shades that enable patients to function best. For Alzheimer's patients, the lighter shades seem to blend together, making it difficult to differentiate a chair from the wall behind it, or the sofa from the floor. Checks, stripes of contrasting colors such as black and white, and polka dots create visual confusion and should be avoided. Simple geometric or repeat designs, plaids, and florals are more welcoming.

Flooring

Next consider flooring. At some point, a patient's gait will become shuffling and perhaps scissorslike. Many patients have a history of falls, and frequently the floor covering is to blame for such mishaps. Care partners should adapt the floor surfaces to accommodate the afflicted person's needs. Before altering the flooring, however, start by checking his footwear — especially if he walks with a "shuffling" gait.

You will probably want to continue to use whatever flooring you already have. But if a room has tile floors, for instance, do not spend time trying to get the perfect shine; cleanliness with a dull finish is fine. Shininess or glare tends to create an illusion of water, ice, or other fear-provoking mirages. Wall-to-wall carpeting, without scatter or area rugs, offers a uniform, secure walking surface, but spills and maintenance may present a problem.

Light-colored carpeting is best, since it tends to make a space seem larger and less confining. Since scatter or area rugs often cause accidents, eliminating them is a good idea for safety. Always be mindful, too, of shadows that may be created on flooring, and adjust window coverings or lights to eliminate the sometimes terrifying visual illusions that can form in the perception of a person with Alzheimer's. For safety's sake, repair or level uneven flooring.

If you have the opportunity to choose new flooring, the ideal surface is a simulated hardwood floor (it can be found in most large home improvement centers), because it is reminiscent of older homes and is easy to care for. It is the first choice of interior designers and architects who build facilities for memory-impaired people.

Interior Pathways

Establishing clear interior pathways will help the person with Alzheimer's negotiate spaces safely. He will also feel a sense of accomplishment at being able to find important places — the bathroom, kitchen, or even a favorite chair — more easily.

Consider placing a colorful wallpaper border at waist height along the walls in the rooms where the patient will be spending time. Unsafe entries and exits can be camouflaged by continuing the border across doors and on the surrounding walls. To someone with failing perception, the doors then seem to be just part of the walls.

In a care facility, scenes or designs can be painted on doors to help deceive the residents while ensuring their safety. Bright thematic borders, such as cactus and tumbleweed for Texas, cornfields for Oklahoma, and so forth, can direct residents to activity rooms, while colorful arrows can show the way to the bathroom. An awning hangs over the entrance to the dining room in one of my favorite facilities.

Furniture and Hangings

Remove furniture that is difficult to get into and out of. As the person's motor skills diminish, balance becomes more tenuous. She will require sturdy chairs with arms to push up from and seats with short depth from front to back. Large, overstuffed furniture can prove difficult for the person with Alzheimer's. A glider is a wonderful addition at this time, both for comfort and for recalling memories of rocking chairs. Unlike rocking chairs, which can be quite hazardous, gliders do not actually lift off the floor — just the seat slides to and fro, providing safe hours of enjoyable rocking. Also, recognize that to someone with changed senses, large pieces of furniture that wobble or move when touched, even if safe, may appear ready to topple. Built-in shelves are always safer and less threatening than freestanding units, and they help to keep areas clutter-free and simplified, thus increasing safety and reducing the sense of being threatened.

Simplicity is the watchword for any item that hangs on a wall. For instance, at some point in the middle stage of the disease, mirrors do more harm than good. A glance in the mirror may make the Alzheimer's person believe that another person is in the room — someone who has not been invited, an intruder, someone who is there to do harm. Because the image seems vaguely familiar, the person may perceive it to be an older, possibly deceased relative — a mother, perhaps, or a father who passed away long ago. This can cause great distress and frustration to someone who can't separate facts of existence from unreality. When you first become aware that the patient is no longer using a mirror to inspect his image, replace it with a different wall decoration. (The same principle holds true for hand-held mirrors or those that rest on surfaces, of course.)

You should think carefully about other wall hangings, too. The cognitively impaired adult can easily misinterpret photographs and pictures on the wall, especially if they are protected by glass. Replace reflective glass with no-glare glass to help the patient focus on the painting or photo and not on what might be generated in her mind from shadows and reflections. Remove images that are abstract or show complicated scenes. Instead, simple pictures of flowers, children, and animals evoke harmonious memories. Textured wall hangings and ones that can be touched, including quilted shams, are a source of great enjoyment. Children's artwork and unframed needlepoint images hung on walls can serve as tactile or conversational pieces.

Faux windows with views of, say, a Maine lighthouse or California coastline can break up stretches of blank wall. Patients react to these "windows" so positively that many such scenes are being created solely for use in Alzheimer's facilities.

Eliminate reminders of hobbies that the patient can no longer take part in — any activity that requires fine coordination, for example. At the same time, to encourage hobbies that he can still perform, keep the crafts or tools in clear view, perhaps near a favorite chair.

Finally, a piece of "furniture" that you may want to add is a sturdy fish tank, which can provide hours of viewing pleasure and a chance for the patient to be nurturing by feeding the fish. You'll have to establish a feeding schedule so the fish aren't fed too often. And set a comfortable chair in front of the tank — not be-

side it — so the patient can watch the fish. Do not depend on the person with Alzheimer's to set up the viewing arrangement.

Use Images to Replace Words

As directions become more difficult and memory less reliable, use images of items to supplant words. Put a picture of dishes on the door of the cabinet where the dishes are stored, a picture of panties on the front of the underwear drawer, a picture of a toilet on the bathroom door or next to the door if you want to leave the door open, especially at night. Frequently assess the environment to adjust or compensate for changes in the patient.

Safety Devices

Many devices can make a patient's surroundings safer. For instance, at the top and bottom of the stairs, you can install child safety gates. Keeping a person with Alzheimer's from climbing stairs is as important as protecting her from falling down them.

Closets also present problems. If the closet doors have knobs, you can install childproof locks on them. These locks, which do not have keys, require some finger dexterity to open but they are quite manageable for most care partners and too complicated for someone who is cognitively impaired. Use these locks to prevent the patient from entering any area where harmful substances are stored, where last season's clothes have been placed out of sight, or where you don't want her to explore. You can also employ these locks to secure items such as medical, cleaning, and other supplies in drawers; one unsuccessful attempt to open a drawer is usually enough to keep the patient from trying again.

If your home has a fireplace, you may want to camouflage the opening by placing something colorful inside it, such as a large basket of yarn or a silk flower arrangement. Remove any fireplace screen or door and put it out of sight. Of course, keep matches and other lighting implements well hidden at all times.

If your stove or oven is electric, have someone install a "kill switch" in a place known only to you. Such switches allow the habilitator to use the stove or oven at will but make it impossible for the patient to turn on. If you have a gas stove or oven, consult your local gas company on how to make it tamperproof. The patient should think of the appliance as broken instead of believing that he is unable to make it work. Keep in mind that the afflicted person's physical safety is not the only concern; his feelings of success also count.

Home Areas

Encouraging socialization is an important part of the habilitation approach, and care partners can generate social interaction by placing chairs at angles to one another to signify a place for conversation. A person with Alzheimer's may not be likely to initiate conversation without such clues. And the creation of cozy spaces often makes a patient feel more emotionally comfortable. In a home in which an afflicted person has lived for many years, rearrange furniture to encourage conversation while keeping the arrangement as close to the original pattern as possible. Coziness can be enhanced, for example, by eating meals in the kitchen rather than in a large dining room, or by eating only at one end of the dining table, after making it distinct from the rest of the table. Keep in mind, when entertaining, that large spaces make people with Alzheimer's particularly uncomfortable, especially in social situations.

Of course, at times we all need solitude. Sometimes, in long-term-care settings, staff members believe that patients need to be constantly engaged; but this is no more true for Alzheimer's people than it is for anyone else. No one wants to have every moment filled with activities that may have little meaning to one's past lifestyle; we all need opportunities to be alone, gathering our thoughts, assessing our feelings, and reviewing the past. The patient may have a much stronger perception of the past than of the

present, so offer her many chances to review it happily and comfortably.

Toward this end, you can put a favorite chair in a corner of a room to encourage her to be alone at times when she seems to need quiet and introspection.

Outdoors

Repair cracked, uneven, or potholed pavement, trying to make the surface as level and smooth as possible (but not slick, of course).

Being outdoors and having contact with nature can contribute to the patient's well-being and sense of security. Bird feeders and houses, birdbaths, wind chimes, and colorful windsocks may all be points of interest. If the afflicted person likes gardening, whether the enjoyment is in planting or simply experiencing warm earth running through the fingers, worms and all, create a raised flower bed, about three feet high, so it can be comfortably reached. Plant a few flowers or herbs to make the purpose of the bed visually obvious at eye level. The height also saves patients from strained backs. Parsley, sage, rosemary, and thyme are wonderful choices for an outdoor (or indoor) herb garden because of their wonderful perfume, splendid foliage, and great taste when eaten. Chives have fine stalks and offer a pale purple bloom, and yellow nasturtiums — like the other plants I've mentioned — are harmless if ingested. All are easy to care for and have a sweet aroma and interesting colors. (Patients cannot always distinguish edible from inedible plants, so check with the local poison-control center to ensure that all outdoor plantings and houseplants are safe.)

If you have a good-sized yard, creating paths for the patient to wander along can help his serenity. Plant bright annuals, such as geraniums, impatiens, and marigolds, along the paths. The flowers act as guideposts and keep patients away from areas that are uneven or otherwise problematic. Make sure that the plants and flowers within reach are not poisonous, since people with Alzheimer's often mistake plants for food.

A bench or outdoor chairs placed at the end of a walkway can serve as a social area, and possibly as a deterrent to going beyond the walkway. A sturdy six-foot fence around the yard might also be necessary to keep the Alzheimer's person out of harm's way. A fenced area also provides a respite for the habilitator, who knows that the patient can enjoy the outdoors without danger of wandering away. Choose a fence material that cannot be seen through — solid wood, perhaps, or brick, rather than chainlink; that will lower the chances of the Alzheimer's patient becoming overstimulated by objects beyond the fence, and will also reduce her desire to get to the other side. Planting bushes and seasonal flowers in front of the fencing will reduce or eliminate feelings of imprisonment.

Noise and Sound

Noise is also part of the environment. The patient's ability to hear does not change, but he interprets sounds differently as time goes on. Research has shown that many of the sounds we take for granted actually disturb patients with progressive dementias. The sounds of television, telephones, flushing toilets, running water, radios, doorbells, alarm clocks, and traffic, for example, can be overstimulating and agitating to a person with Alzheimer's.

Monitor the patient for signs that she is not able to understand words or separate sounds or that she is scared of noises. Does the soft whirr of an air conditioner seem to be an ever-present annoyance, no matter how loudly she tries to talk over it? Does she fear that every passing car is going to crash into the house?

Unfortunately, as of this writing, there is no test available to evaluate exactly what sounds the patient is hearing or differentiating. But many early-stage patients have said that they function best in a quiet space, and that they become lost in a conver-

sation if more than one person speaks. Furthermore, two or more sounds occurring at once — a bird singing while a baby laughs, for example — can easily overwhelm a person who is struggling to sort out simple information. And an additional background sound, such as that of a furnace, can truly be confounding, as if the noise is coming from within the patient's own head.

If an unexpected sound frightens the person with Alzheimer's, quickly show him what made the sound and repeat the incident. If a pan drops on a floor, for example, drop it again, and point out that you, too, were shaken by the sound. Of course, it's good to avoid having things fall noisily on a tiled floor, for example, and cause clattering; place a nonslip mat on the floor when doing kitchen chores to cushion the sounds and limit breakage.

Sometimes sounds may be frustrating to a patient by reminding her of her shortcomings. Sounds of a meal being prepared can bring back memories of what she can no longer do. Being aware of and sensitive to this problem will help you discover some ways to solve it. You may be able to arrive at an answer without too much trouble.

For instance, at certain times of the day Elliott noted that Janelle's conversation would get louder and louder. All too often, he said, his wife would shout so strongly that neighbors would come over to see if everything was all right. Elliott was stumped. The commotions did not happen all the time and never after the couple went to bed, even though they often had long conversations about the day's happenings then. Elliott also realized that the shouting occurred only in their home. Clearly, Janelle was trying to speak louder than some bothersome sound she could not identify. Using a behavior log to keep track of this troubling behavior when it happened (see Chapter 9), Elliot uncovered the source of her agitation: the noise of warm air humming through the heating ducts. Elliot was so accustomed to the noise he never noticed it, but Janelle registered the sound as something new, an annoyance that could be overcome only by speaking at the top of her lungs. Elliot called in a heating company to wrap the pipes to deaden the sound. He also installed carpet on the cellar ceiling to further muffle the sounds of the furnace.

If you have an area where noise is particularly bothersome, try installing some temporary acoustical ceiling tiles on the walls. You can place sound-diffusing transparent contact paper on windows if street sounds are an annoyance. And don't hesitate to draw the draperies and turn on lights in broad daylight if that will produce a quieter situation. Textured wall coverings (either paint or wallpaper) can help to diffuse sound.

You can also use noise to enhance the patient's safety. Jingle bells or sleigh bells hung on a door or gate can alert a care partner to an attempt to get out, averting a potentially harmful situation. Some hardware and department stores have "traveler's locks" that hang on a doorknob and emit a shrill sound when the knob is turned.

Research has shown that patients' difficulty processing sounds is upsetting for only a short period during the progression of the disease. Perhaps as the person with Alzheimer's retreats more into her own world, she is bothered less by the noises and acoustical interruptions from the outside world. It is very important, however, to pay attention to what is happening during the period when she feels assaulted by noises and is unable to separate or identify the various sounds.

The $100 Hardware Store Revolution*

- Purchase an emergency power-failure light (less than $15).
- Pick up a hand-held shower (about $25).
- Buy a door alarm (about $40).
- Spend the rest of the $100 on halogen light bulbs and double-sided tape or other skid-proofing for throw rugs.
- Throw in another few dollars and buy a timer for the outdoor lights.

*Courtesy of Jeanette Rosa-Brady of the Massachusetts Alzheimer's Association.

Habilitation requires care partners to think creatively, applying the five tenets to each situation to arrive at resourceful adjustments. Consider the following examples.

Early one morning, Steve looked out his window on the second-floor landing. The day was going to be beautiful. He smiled as he felt the warm sunshine on his face, then he took two steps forward and toppled headfirst down a flight of stairs. An early-stage Alzheimer's patient, Steve was having trouble distinguishing depth and contrast, and he did not see the stairwell's empty space. That afternoon Steve's son, Tom, laid strings of white Christmas lights against the wall along one side of the stairs, outlining each step, and installed an overhead light to illuminate the stairwell. A timer automatically turned on all the lights at three P.M. and shut them off at nine A.M. Tom also painted the stairwell yellow to contrast with the white walls of the upstairs hall. Tom smoothly altered the environment to solve a potentially hazardous situation without resorting to safety gates or moving Steve to a downstairs room.

Lois's problem was more difficult for her care partner to pin down. One day she stood in the middle of her living room, staring at the floor, for over an hour. Her husband, Ron, begged her to sit down or come to the den. Each time he spoke, Lois looked up and seemed to see him for the first time. Then she quickly looked down again. Ron finally realized that Lois was dealing with an overload of visual information. Standing amid piles of familiar, memory-laden objects, knitting magazines, and photographs, she could not decide where to sit or what to do. Ron discarded unneeded items and cleared off table surfaces. He replaced standard lamp bulbs with bulbs that mimicked sunlight and hung new, sheer curtains to replace the worn blinds. (The late afternoon sun had cast frightening shadows across the walls.) Leaving a space beside Lois's favorite chair where several mementos and her knitting bag could have the place of honor, he threw a bright afghan over the back of the chair to draw Lois's attention to it. Finally, anticipating problems to come, Ron painted the

front door and trim the same color as the walls to help camouflage the exit. Utilizing just a handful of habilitation techniques,
Ron made it possible for Lois to enjoy her knitting and other
daily tasks for the first time in a long time.

One day Sean, who was having memory problems, tried to call
his sister, just as he did every day. But the woman who answered
was not Annie; he had dialed the wrong number. He dialed again
and got a telephone company recording. Realizing that he had
been unable to recall her telephone number four times in as many
weeks, he sat in his chair, looking at the telephone. Finally it rang,
startling him. His sister, who had recognized that something
must be wrong with Sean, was on the line. The next day Annie
bought him a new telephone with oversized buttons. She pro-
grammed each button with Sean's most important telephone
numbers and replaced the numerals with a photograph or symbol: Annie's picture on 1, Sean's best friend on 2, an ambulance
on 3, and the image of a hypodermic needle (for Sean's physician)
on 4, and so on.

Like the care partners in the above scenarios, you will not need
to incorporate every one of the recommendations in this chapter.
But a few simple adaptations will make the home safer and more
habilitative, a setting where the patient and family can thrive.
Don't hesitate to be creative — the issues will vary from patient
to patient and from day to day, and they will have to be revisited
often as the disease progresses. Making the most of the surroundings will maximize the Alzheimer's person's abilities.

7

Tenet #2: Know That
Communication Remains Possible

You are smiling at me.
I see my reflection in your eyes.
I've finally found someone
who speaks my language.

REMEMBER THAT the emotions behind failing words are far more important than the words themselves and it is the emotions that need to be validated. Although many losses occur with this disease, assume that the patient can still register feelings that matter.

Difficulties with Language

"Shut," Stacey screamed at her husband with her hands held tightly over her ears. "Shut, shut, shut!"

Russell had no idea what he had done to elicit this angry response from his usually soft-spoken wife. He crossed the room to where she was standing and gently enfolded her in his arms, letting her sob gently against his chest. It seemed like such a short time ago that Stacey had gone from having difficulty finding words to making up words to struggling to say anything.

"I've been talking too much, haven't I, Stacey? You want me to just shut up, and I don't blame you." Her husband understood that she was struggling, and as her comprehension declined, that the inability to communicate was becoming unbearable. Angrily placing her hands over her ears and yelling "Shut" was her way of letting Russell know she was overwhelmed by his talking. Even though words failed her, her emotion came through loud and clear.

Difficulties with language often cause emotional outbursts such as Stacey's. We must always look for human emotions and qualities that are being repressed but are ready to burst free when the afflicted person wants to make a statement.

Imagine the anguish of having your ability to talk with loved ones, chat with friends, and exchange greetings with strangers slowly taken away from you. Imagine the frustration of thinking you are saying something clearly, then realizing that the person you're addressing does not understand a single word coming out of your mouth. Imagine, too, listening to someone speaking to you and not being sure what language she is using. This is the reality of life for people with Alzheimer's.

In the early stage of the disease, speech problems range from occasional word-finding difficulties to a profound loss of language. Then the ability to process and store information declines. Clinicians agree that in the middle stage a "verbal casserole" becomes common, with disconnected thoughts spoken aloud and invented words and sounds replacing real ones. In the final stage of the disease, speech all but disappears. Throughout the process, the emotional toll on both patient and care partner is enormous.

Reading and writing abilities also change, and for some patients, following a story line becomes impossible. With diminishing attention, memory, and comprehension and declining ability to think logically, understand metaphors and idioms, and make one's needs known, many people with progressive dementias become silent. They do not wish to make verbal errors, and they're frustrated knowing what they want to say and being unable to say it. They become agitated when we do not take the time to figure out the message or when they see negativity or hopelessness in our eyes.

Often the patient will misuse, bastardize, or alter familiar words altogether. Get to know the patterns and be sure to explain any important "words" to other care partners watching over the person with Alzheimer's, even if only temporarily. My husband, for example, used the word "smish" for sandwich. After a while, "smish" meant "food," and he would say "smish" whenever he was hungry.

Remember that in the person with Alzheimer's, the way the brain processes outside stimuli physically changes. Although you are clearly saying, for example, "I bought some lamb chops. Would you like one for dinner?" he may be hearing, "Wooden lamps are dimmer" — and wonder why you are repeating yourself and seem to be waiting for a reply.

If the person doesn't seem to understand you, break down your sentences into less complex patterns, establish eye contact when possible, and use simple, short statements to alleviate the stress related to failing communication. Remember that processing language will take longer than before — give the person time to think. At some point, the processing mechanism may fail completely. The patient just won't understand what's said.

To further complicate matters, when a person with Alzheimer's is word-searching or using clearly incorrect words, he or she may still be able to understand spoken language. Similarly, a patient who is speaking fairly well may have great difficulty comprehending what is being said.

The upshot is that you should always assume that the person understands language and is included in any dialogue. Even if she appears uninterested or bored, speaks out at inappropriate times, or is not speaking logically, continue to show her that she is valued and is still a part of social or family life. A chief complaint of early-stage patients is not being included in conversations.

People with Alzheimer's often complain that others ignore them in conversations — intentionally or unintentionally. Outsiders who do not include the person in conversation often assume that it is no longer worth talking to the patient. This problem may begin when the doctor gives the initial diagnosis. A couple I know were with their doctor, going over the husband's test results. The doctor looked up and said, "Well, Cristina, I think you need to take Jason on that vacation you've both been waiting for. There's a possibility you won't be able to travel too much longer. I'm sorry to say it, but it looks like Jason has dementia of the Alzheimer's type."

At this juncture, Jason stood up and, banging his fist on the doctor's desk, said, "Damn it all. Am I invisible? This is *my* disease you're talking about — I'm still here. Talk to me. Me!"

The doctor apologized, looked directly into Jason's face, and told him, "Your diagnosis is most probably Alzheimer's disease. Most of the tests point in that direction. Let's do another MRI scan in six months and compare it with the one you took last week. Does that sound logical?"

"Yes," Jason said. "Thank you for telling me."

Communication difficulties may begin at the same time as other problems, making the situation even more difficult. For the person experiencing cognitive decline, the slow loss of coherent speech will be compounded by a declining ability to draw conclusions.

"It is so cold," Nancy said, gazing out the window. "And it's raining so hard outside." At that point, her husband, Douglas, nodded at her, roused himself from the chair where he been sitting for the past few hours, and proceeded out the front door without putting on any kind of raingear. For Douglas, the cause-and-effect thinking that the rest of us practice subconsciously every day no longer existed. The last word he heard Nancy utter was "outside," so he followed that verbal cue, with no thought of protecting himself from the elements.

Many care partners tell me they use this "last-word connection" to their advantage. They relate that this technique actually can help a person with Alzheimer's feel in control of decision-making. Here's how the technique works. The care partner asks, "Would you like to wear this green shirt today, or the one that's blue?" Nine times out of ten, the patient says, "Blue" — simply because it was the last word he remembered hearing. If you ask, "For lunch today, do you want a tuna fish sandwich or cheese?" the response will be "cheese." The wonderfully habilitative part of this technique is that the afflicted person, who is prone to feelings of failure or defeat, now feels able to make choices.

Emotional Communication: Beyond Words

Words are only one part of communication, of course. When visiting an Alzheimer's unit in a long-term-care facility, I frequently come across small groups or pairs of people relating to each other as dear old friends. They appear to be reliving more youthful times and laughing together as they share stories of their past. Upon closer inspection, I sometimes find that each person is speaking a different language, perhaps the foreign language he or she grew up with. Yet even with no words in common, the emotional communication takes place.

I can only assume that Alzheimer's patients focus on the speaker's eyes and determine meaning through tone and gestures, much the way we can watch television without the sound on and still understand the plot. In the same way, if your boss has ever instructed you to come into her office and then has proceeded to take a telephone call, you don't need any words to tell you how she really feels about you.

Everyone uses gestures and pictures, tone and voice pitch, facial expressions and body movements, to convey messages to friends, colleagues, family, and strangers. At times, body language seems more honest and reliable than words. People with Alzheimer's, in trying to compensate for their cognitive and sensory losses, pay more attention to this nonverbal communication and become quite adept at understanding it.

Consider a situation in which I found myself three decades ago. I was trying to direct my husband to sit in a chair. Several attempts had failed, and I felt close to the breaking point at the end of a long day. I had helped with fourth-grade homework, made brownies, diapered and rediapered a toddler, and now this.

"Just do it because I love you," I said in a flat tone.

He immediately stepped close to me and placed his forefinger gently on my eyes. "No," he said clearly and, touching my eyes again, repeated, "No." And he was right. At the moment that I was declaring love, my eyes denied the words. In his own way, he was saying loudly and clearly, "Your eyes don't love me."

Whenever you need the person with Alzheimer's to complete a task, you will be able to communicate your message in far less time by showing patience and confidence through body language as well as words. As we've seen in the context of dining and bathing, taking time to sit with the patient, to talk about simple things without expecting a response, is one of the best ways to win cooperation. Communication says that we value the patient. Also, never underestimate the power of physical communication with a person who has Alzheimer's. Touch is a marvelous expression of nurturing and security.

Here are some specific guidelines for communicating positively:

- Approach the person in a calm, gentle way, and always from the front, to foster trust.
- Set the stage for discourse with a tone that reflects respect.
- Speak slowly, in a low tone, using simple sentences rather than complicated language patterns. The patient's hearing is not the problem, so raising your voice is not the answer.

• Be patient; the person with progressive dementia takes extra time to process information.

When people other than family members are going to be with the patient, be sure to tell them about his personal vocabulary, so that they use familiar terms for any concepts they are trying to communicate. If the last meal of the day has always been referred to as "dinner," then calling the patient to "supper" will not achieve the expected response.

Use simple language, because idioms, metaphors, slang, and other speech variations are extremely difficult for a person with Alzheimer's to interpret. If you suggest to a patient that she is "pulling my leg," be prepared for her to literally do just that.

When you need to have a serious conversation, find a quiet place where the patient will not be overstimulated. The best place is one where you can sit at right angles to the patient, establish eye contact, and hopefully touch him to show your support, concern, and love during the conversation.

Assure the patient frequently that her communication is successful. She knows failure all too well and needs constant reassurance that she is still a functioning human being. When the patient's words are mixed up and seem nonsensical, smile, touch her, and simply say, "I am having a problem understanding." This underscores that she is not the problem.

Avoid asking open-ended questions. Statements are preferable because they do not call upon the person to make decisions. "Let's have a cup of coffee" will reap a response, while "Do you want a cup of coffee?" may garner a "no" when, in fact, he or she would love coffee but can no longer verbalize the choice. "No" often seems the safer reply to a question. A person with Alzheimer's is likely to perceive questions as a kind of testing, which makes him feel like a failure.

Humor remains the best way to communicate. Laughing at oneself is a true gift; laughing with someone else is the greatest joy. Watch comedy videotapes together, listen to humorous audio cassettes, and read aloud funny anecdotes. Often it is the laughter itself that brings pleasure; the patient doesn't necessarily have to understand the punch line. Recall amusing situations you have shared, and laugh together until your sides hurt.

Remember the power of music, a universal tool for communicating with those whose language is impaired. A Mozart flute concerto speaks to people from many countries and backgrounds; people of all ages and many ethnicities clap along to a Sousa march. Ethnic and religious music can be used to lull someone to sleep, to encourage recall, and to calm obstreperous behavior. Of particular therapeutic value is the music from a person's early cultural background. And many people with progressive dementias who are described as nonverbal can still sing every word of "Happy Birthday." (The best Alzheimer's programs employ a music therapist as a permanent staff member to reach nonverbal residents through song and dance, exercise, and reminiscing.)

Always listen to the emotion behind the patient's failing words. The emotion is still intact; at some elemental level, you can still reach it. The actual words are not important if you can understand the feeling behind the attempt to communicate.

8

Tenet #3:
Focus on Remaining Skills

I suffer most for my loss
of self-esteem,
not for the loss
of choosing my wardrobe.

Focus only on the skills that the patient still has. Value whatever abilities remain. Help her compensate for any lost abilities without bringing them to her attention.

Those of us without dementia can go through our activities of daily living without thinking or rehearsal. While other thoughts occupy our minds, we shower, dress, eat breakfast, listen to the morning news, tie a Windsor knot, fasten jewelry, and take on the day. That's not true for Alzheimer's patients, of course.

Bathing

Of all the activities of daily living, the biggest single problem for most care partners appears to be keeping an Alzheimer's patient clean. Why, adult children wonder, does Father want to be dirty all of a sudden? Why does Mom refuse to take a shower? A wife can't understand why her husband behaves like a lion when faced with a washcloth; a husband is frustrated when his wife screams when she looks into the bubbles of a warm bath.

Unfortunately, the battle of the bath begins early in the disease process and, without the habilitation approach, continues till the end. Consider the scene Paulette and her health-care aide, Jayne, had during one bath time. Jayne had been trying to coax Paulette, who exhibited most of the typical signs of the middle stage of Alzheimer's, into the tub for almost twenty minutes. Paulette was standing beside the bathtub shivering; the towel wrapped around her midsection did little to warm her or to protect whatever vanity remained.

"Just get into the nice bath," pleaded Jayne. "You haven't had a good bath in days."

Paulette, who had limited language use, first replied, "Go, go, wo, wo, wo." Then she started talking louder and began shaking her fist at the mirror.

Tired of the battle, Jayne leaned over slightly to lift one of Paulette's feet into the warm water.

"No, no, no," Paulette screamed, suddenly pummeling and scratching at Jayne's face and arms. "No, no, no!"

Jayne gave up and took Paulette back to her bedroom.

Every day, thousands of patients and care partners in homes and facilities go through this kind of battle. In most cases, the habilitation approach can ameliorate the situation.

Although I have stated this before, it is well worth repeating: *Never attempt to reason with someone who has lost her reason.* Twenty minutes was far too long a time for Jayne to try to coax Paulette into a bath. A long discussion about the need for a shower or bath will lead only to confrontation and a fractured ego. And Paulette's fear, suspicion, and chills must have grown during the course of the standoff.

What's more, Jayne should have kept Paulette thoroughly wrapped until she stepped into the bath. A care partner should remove the warming garment at the last moment, even if that means getting the edges of it wet. Clothes and towels dry quickly — spirits take far longer to heal. Jayne should also have removed the mirror from the bathroom, since it's very likely that Paulette became even more distressed by the perception of an additional person in the room.

Next, Jayne needed to be more attentive to Paulette's emotions, taking the time to reassure her and to establish trust. For example, Jayne could have chatted about a topic of interest to Paulette while making the bath preparations, letting Paulette feel that she was involved in the process.

When Jayne leaned in front of Paulette, she would have been much safer if she had first given the patient a washcloth to hold and focus on. Paulette would then not have had time to be afraid or worried. Intimidation and fear are generally the triggers for malevolent behavior during bathing time. Resistance is not a conscious choice — the patient truly does not have the cognitive powers to make the decision to fight.

Several problems may crop up each time a person with Alzheimer's faces a bath or shower:

- The patient may perceive the bath or shower as a first-time ordeal every time. He simply may not remember the expectations of bath time.
- Removing clothing — or having it removed — can increase feelings of loss of control. The inability to articulate those feelings can raise the patient's anxiety.
- The sound of running water may induce fear in someone with failing auditory perception.
- Impaired perception of color, depth, and contrast may keep the patient from seeing clear water. Adding a blue or blue-green coloring agent to the tub helps make the water visible.
- The feeling of water suddenly splashed on the face can cause fear. If possible, wash the patient's face and hands separately,

not in the shower. Shampooing can also cause anxiety, so shampoo only when you must do so, and use dry shampoo whenever possible.

• The odor of an unfamiliar kind of soap may induce fear.

The person's shortened attention span may cause another problem. Don't ever suggest that the patient "wait a minute" while you get something ready. One woman in a care-partner support group told us how she had her husband all prepared for his shower when she realized she had forgotten fresh towels. "That's when the fateful 'wait a minute' escaped my lips," she said. "I went to get the towels and he went for a walk, stark naked, out the front door." Her husband simply did not have a long enough attention span to wait.

The habilitator trying to instill confidence should maximize the creature comforts. Light a lavender-scented candle, offer a soothing cup of tea or glass of wine (be sure the cup or glass is plastic, however). And why not play some soft background music? The bathroom should be warm, well lit, and have nonskid rugs and safety bars. Place a shower chair in the stall or use a bath bench (see Further Resources, page 226) in the tub, close the shades or curtains, and shut the door. If you are giving the patient a shower, use a hand-held nozzle and work from the feet up. This method gives the person a chance to feel the water's warmth and a sense of pleasure as the water slowly moves up his body.

If you know that the person you are helping will become anxious — as Paulette did — give her something other than the bath to focus on. Along with washcloths, sponges and loofas work well. One care partner I know placed a lava lamp nearby to capture her husband's attention while she gave him a scrub.

If a bath or shower causes panic, try giving just a sponge bath. Sequencing the steps will help keep the patient as involved as possible. First, with the patient wrapped in a terrycloth robe or towel, you might say, "Hmm, this is a nice warm cloth." Wait a moment, then hand it to her, saying, "Wash your face." Have a towel ready and, when she is done, let her dry her face herself. Then move on to the next body part, exposing only whatever is necessary. Offer simple instructions, demonstrate with gestures, and show that you are not in a hurry. Offer praise whenever possible, of course.

Giving a bath may require some real ingenuity on your part. My friend Susan gave new meaning to the term "sponge bath" when her husband, Tyler, made it quite clear that he was never going to bathe again. A six-foot-four-inch-tall career marine, Tyler one day underscored his determination by picking up his five-foot-two wife and plunking her down on top of the washing machine in their townhouse. Tyler's language had failed considerably, and he rarely spoke, but Susan understood what he meant. Determined to find a way to get her husband clean, this feisty woman, equipped with a pail of warm sudsy water, waited for Tyler to fall into his "snoring stage" of sleep each night, and then she got out her sponge and started to work.

If he began to wake up, she said, "I would throw a towel over him, pull up the covers, and run like hell. He never ever caught me, and he was relatively clean from then on. Boy, was I proud. It took four days to get his whole body clean and then I'd start again. But he never caught on." That was creative care partnering.

Dressing

Outsiders often perceive a patient's careless or sloppy dressing as showing a lack of interest, when it actually may just be the inability to cope with buttons, zippers, snaps, or jewelry, all of which require considerable finger dexterity. Having put together a fairly unconventional ensemble by herself, the patient may feel well dressed. But she may register the care partner's expression of embarrassment, anger, or frustration. And later in the disease, when the patient certainly requires assistance with dressing, how a care partner does this can affect the patient's emotions for several days.

Consider the patient's reactions in these two situations, which were discussed in one support group.

Scott was filling the dishwasher with the breakfast cutlery as Beverly came down the front stairs ready for her Saturday morning hairdresser appointment. Scott finished up, stepped around the corner, and looked at his wife.

"What the heck do you think you're doing?" he said.

His response took Beverly aback. "What do you mean?"

"Look at how you're dressed. Now go back upstairs and put on the right clothes. And hurry up or we'll be late."

Beverly went back up to her room, lowered herself onto the edge of the bed, and waited for some time. Scott's voice broke her reverie. "Beverly, are you ready? We have to go right this minute or we'll be too late. C'mon, let's go — now."

Beverly gathered her pocketbook and started down the front stairs, hoping that Scott would already be in the car and that they could avoid another confrontation. But when she stepped outside, Scott saw her and jumped out of the car. He raced toward her, grabbing her arm, and hurriedly ushered her back inside the house.

"Ow! Scott," Beverly whimpered. "What did I do? Why do you hate me?"

"I don't know why you are doing this to me! I can't take you anywhere dressed like this. For cripe's sake, those are your gardening pants, and that's the blouse you wore to the Valentine's Day dance at the club. All the people at the salon are going to think you're nuts — or that I am, for letting you go out like that."

Beverly ended up in bed in tears, with Scott phoning the salon to cancel her appointment.

Contrast that scene with another scenario. One Thursday, as was their custom, Jan took her mother, Melanie, to a local seafood restaurant for a four o'clock "early-bird special." It was raining, and Jan was late picking up her mother. Melanie was already bundled up and ready to go.

When they reached the restaurant, the maitre d' showed them

to their table, and Jan suggested that Melanie remove her coat. When she did, there she was in all her glory, clothed only in a thin, well-worn pink slip, with one strap held up with a tiny gold safety pin.

Jan's response was the best way to turn what could have been a humiliating catastrophe for both mother and daughter into a seemingly normal evening with no loss of self-esteem. She leaned across the table and said, "It's so chilly in here tonight that I'm keeping my coat on — how about you?" Her mother nodded in agreement, and let a blushing young waiter help her back into her wrap.

When I asked Jan if she had been horribly embarrassed, she replied that she felt the situation wasn't about her — it was about maintaining her mother's dignity. That night Jan and Melanie's dinner was lovely, as always. The experience underscored a habilitation lesson: it isn't Alzheimer's that takes away the person's dignity; it's other people's reactions that do.

Think about how the situation with Beverly and Scott could have been improved. "That blouse is so beautiful," he could have said, "I think you should save it for when we go out to dinner tonight. And how about if I find your sweater that's brown, the one that goes so nicely with those slacks, which are brown?" (Repeating the word "brown" and ending the sentence with "brown" would make Beverly more likely to remember it.)

And if Beverly had resisted the change of clothing, the worst-case scenario would have found her at the beauty salon decked out in an odd outfit — but that probably wouldn't have bothered the hairdresser, who must have already noticed the changes in Beverly's behavior. Every care partner needs to smile tolerantly at a few odd fashion statements if she is going to survive. Remember whose problem it is — and whose dignity you are trying to save.

After Scott brought up Beverly's dressing problem in his support group, he figured out how he could better handle such situations in the future. Scott asked his daughter to come over and begin weeding out Beverly's closet. Along with making sure that only seasonal outfits remained, the daughter hung matching pieces together, choosing as many solid colors as possible. When Beverly noticed that some of her clothes were missing, Scott mentioned that the garments were in storage — a "fiblet" that brought peace.

Several weeks later the daughter returned to remove a few more items, and she kept doing so until the closet contained only those clothes that would complement each other. Although Beverly's clothes choices would not make her look the way she used to before her diagnosis, they were reasonably appropriate. Most important, she could feel a sense of control in her world.

How to Help a Patient Dress Successfully

Choose clothing for:

- Ease. The garment can be put on and taken off easily.
- Comfort. The clothing does not restrict movement.
- Recognizability. Try to use clothing that the patient can easily recognize. Buy the same outfit again and again; if it wears out or is too stained, you know it is a favorite.
- Familiarity. Do not introduce new styles or faddish clothes.
- Color. Choose colors that you know the patient will enjoy or would have chosen for himself.
- Touch. Use textured clothing when you can. Velvet and silks are lovely to touch.

Here are some clothing choices that have proved to be useful:

- Simple, comfortable socks and shoes
- Slip-on, Velcro-tabbed shoes or sneakers
- Ankle-high socks (all the same color and type, to avoid mismatches and reduce anxiety)
- Knee-high stockings for women
- Open-collar shirts and dresses
- Clothes that are one size larger than usual
- Shirts and dresses that pull on over the head
- Elastic-waist, loose-fitting pants
- Avoid clothes that have zippers or buttons, are tight or otherwise restrictive, or confuse the patient.

Never act as if you're in a hurry if you need to assist a patient dressing. A person with Alzheimer's disease needs considerably more time to process information and can usually handle only one command at a time.

Try to schedule appointments in the afternoon whenever possible. When you have no alternative to an early schedule, be sure to set out the afflicted person's clothes the night before, so they are ready to be put on in the morning.

Other problems may also make an Alzheimer's patient unable to dress as she used to. Muriel, for example, was in the late-middle stage of Alzheimer's and, much to her sister Nina's chagrin, she wore the same yellow dress day after day. Sometimes Muriel even wore the dress to bed. And she often wanted to wear it when shopping with Nina; no amount of cajoling or reasoning changed Muriel's mind. Probably Muriel wasn't aware that the dress was soiled and wrinkled, since she was no longer sensitive to hygiene and tidiness.

Nina could have found a way to bypass this common situation. She could wait until Muriel was asleep, remove the yellow dress, and then buy several similar dresses that offered the same simplicity and comfort and color that made the dress so appealing to Muriel.

And don't worry about buying clothing that you would not have purchased for the patient in the past. Although you may never have imagined your mother in a sweatsuit, for example, the time may come when such a suit is the most comfortable way to dress, particularly in the late stage of the disease.

A problem that crops up with many people who have Alzheimer's is wanting to undress at inappropriate times. For the patient who loves to disrobe, the answer can be a one-piece jumpsuit with a zipper in the back. Or you can give the person a "busy apron" to distract him when he tries to remove his clothes. A busy apron is nothing more than a regular apron with many items sewn onto it — for example, buttons, zippers, ribbon, flowers, dangling objects, keys, and so on. It keeps the patient's hands engaged and minimizes frustration. (The Products section of Further Resources, page 223, lists suppliers of comfortable clothing and useful gadgets.)

You may also find that when a woman requires assistance with grooming and dressing, you can help her by applying a little fragrance or makeup, even if she has never used such niceties before. When outsiders pass her in the supermarket or the corridor of the nursing home, they may smile or compliment her.

Similarly, don't forget the value of complimenting a patient on his looks. Complimenting someone with progressive dementia may not only add to feelings of self-worth, but, as inhibitions dissipate with the progress of the disease, may result in an effusive affirmative reaction. Stephanie shared with her support group what happened when she complimented her shy father, who was dressed in his "usual navy suit." Her comment, "You look really great today, Dad," resulted in his sweeping her up in a bear hug, and suddenly involving her in a two-step dance around the living room. Stephanie said she had never felt so close to her father; her compliment and his response were the beginning of a new phase in their relationship.

Eating

Care partners often become frustrated when soup cascades down a patient's shirt front, fingers end up gloved in bright orange squash, or coffee swims over mashed potatoes on a plate. This is what was upsetting Fran when she called me about her father. "From now on I am going to feed him myself," she said. "I can't take it anymore. He was always so well groomed. He'd die if he knew what he looked like now — covered with food. And he runs the other way when he sees me."

Fran needed to learn that the goal is not impeccable social dining skills but — at this point you know the answer — as much independence as possible. The biggest challenge for care partners is in adjusting their attitude, accepting the patient as he is now, not expecting him to be who he once was. Fran was projecting her disdain onto her father, with the result that he actually ran the other way when she approached him.

Patients can have trouble dining for several reasons, including the following:

- Inability to recognize how items are used
- Failing visual perception
- Diminishing attention span
- Language difficulties
- Declining motor skills
- Reduced social graces

Introduce finger foods when the patient is in the early stages of the disease, before the need becomes imperative. Finger foods are the best choice for maintaining dignity, providing opportunities for success, and encouraging proper nutrition. Such foods don't require utensils, condiments, or plates and can be served at any time of day as snacks or at regular mealtimes. Finger foods can be served throughout most of the disease process. (See the Appendix, page 207, for finger food suggestions.)

In the example below, see if you can identify habilitative methods that would improve the outcome. (Coming up with answers for at least six problems will earn you an A.)

At Jameson and Louise's small dining table, Jameson set the radio so he could listen to a football game. Louise laid a flowered place mat on the striped tablecloth and set the table with silverware and a plate. Next she brought in the teapot, sugar bowl, creamer, salt and pepper shakers, and a carefully folded napkin. She set a white porcelain bowl of fruit in the middle of the table. For years the couple had used this arrangement for their meals. Jameson would listen to sports games at the table, while Louise would carry her plate to the den and watch television as she ate.

Louise next brought out a large bowl of macaroni and cheese and set it in front of her husband, saying, "Try not to make too much of a mess." As she walked away, she heard a crash. She turned around and saw Jameson half standing, with the macaroni bowl and the food at his feet. What's more, he was eating a bright orange tangerine — peel and all.

What could have been changed to make the experience easier for both Jameson and Louise? First, Louise should have turned off the radio. Mealtime is the wrong time for extra sound, with Jameson needing every grain of his remaining attention capability to focus on eating. And the time of the meal could be changed so he could listen to the game later, since it was such a source of enjoyment for him.

Setting a place mat on the tablecloth provided too much visual stimulation for Jameson. The different patterns created a sense of visual bombardment. The best choice is a mat that contrasts with the table and with the plate, to aid both visual contrast and depth perception. For example, on a wooden table, use a solid-color mat and a white plate: the plate will contrast with the mat, which in turn contrasts with the table; the food will be the primary focus of attention.

Jameson never noticed the macaroni and cheese, which in his simplified color palette matched the white bowl. Louise could have put the mainly white food on a brightly contrasting plate. Or she could have shaken some red paprika on top of the food, or chopped chives, ketchup, or grated yellow cheese. (These tricks also work for white vegetables, such as cauliflower, and fish.)

Louise should have put out only the silverware Jameson would need for the food she was serving. All the silverware created an additional stimulant for him. Just a soup spoon or tablespoon would have been fine for the macaroni and cheese, given Jameson's declining motor skills. Serving a sandwich would have been even better, since then Jameson would not have needed any utensils. (According to the same habilitative principle, the best way to present soup is in a mug.)

Like many people with Alzheimer's, Jameson could not distinguish the edible part of the fruit from the inedible skin. One day I searched for a missing banana, only to learn, hours later, that the patient I was working with had devoured it, peel and all; another time he ate a tea bag. Fruit should be kept out of sight or peeled and left out as a handy "help-yourself" snack. Frequent small meals might have been better for Jameson if he had a short attention span. Leaving easily spotted, nutritious finger foods in various places can help a person with progressive dementia get the nutrition he needs.

Finally, Louise's derogatory remark about a mess did nothing to boost Jameson's feelings of self-esteem. Even when cleaning up after a mishap, a care partner using the habilitation approach tries to avoid making the person with Alzheimer's feel responsible for the problem. The day will come when you no longer have to deal with accidents and calamities. Believe it or not, you may miss them.

Eating, of course, is not just a matter of physical skills but also a question of nutritional intake. The care partner needs to monitor changes in the patient's weight and eating habits, evaluating whether the alteration may be the result of a physical or medical condition. Can the patient say that she is cold or thirsty? Does she recognize food as the answer to hunger?

Stay on the lookout for possible dehydration, which may occur because the patient no longer recognizes the signal of thirst, because she is taking certain medications, or because she is simply not drinking enough fluids. You should offer fluids throughout the day, but not after supper, to discourage urination at night. If you notice that the person with Alzheimer's seems to be losing weight, check for ill-fitting dentures or aching teeth. He may not be able to report such problems, which might make eating more difficult.

What if the person doesn't seem to be hungry at mealtime? To stir up an appetite and bring the mind around to thoughts of mealtime, offer a bit of wine or grape juice in a cocktail glass before dinner. The only snacks offered before meals should be a healthful selection of sliced vegetables and a dip to take the place of a vegetable served during the meal.

Recognize that large portions can easily overwhelm the patient, even if big servings pleased him in the past. Tastes also change, and at some point you may need to augment food with condiments, herbs, and spices for someone with progressive dementia. You may be able to encourage the patient to eat by adding a little sugar to the food, even if she previously didn't care for sweets. Many care partners sprinkle brown sugar on scrambled eggs and mix softened chocolate chips into whipped potatoes. These combinations may not be to our taste, but we're not the ones with the disease.

If the patient is reluctant to take medications, you can in many cases purchase the medicines in liquid form and blend them into an appealing shake (see the Appendix, page 210, for blender recipes). Shakes are a good way to provide additional nutrients when the person is not eating well.

Sometimes the person with Alzheimer's simply needs a visual cue to start eating. A quiet table for two is a good setting for engaging the patient in the social ritual of eating. Eat with her whenever you can, for the need for human interaction is constant. What's more, some social graces may surface when least expected. The afflicted person may be only a passive conversational partner, but you can chat about pleasant happenings in the world or your life. You can talk about books, movies, sports, or fashions, even though the discussion will not be what it was before the impairment. And, as a bonus, dining together is an opportunity for the patient to mimic your dining style — a built-in cueing system without words but with a positive use of body language.

Whether or not you eat with the patient, make sure that the lighting is good enough to focus clearly on the meal, yet not so bright as to cast shadows, which can be disruptive. As I've mentioned, shadows may elicit hallucinations or raise the level of the patient's stress.

It is a good idea to cover the patient's clothing to keep spills from becoming a problem, but don't use a childish bib. Cover yourself the same way you cover the patient and say, "This may be a messy meal for both of us," as you spread the lap towel. To avoid confusion, serve no more than one item at a time. You might put a mug of soup in front of the patient, then remove the mug when she has finished, before bringing in a sandwich.

If you are the care partner but not a family member, find out about the patient's favorite foods and accustomed dining schedule from someone who knows her more personally. Ask when she eats the day's biggest meal. Learn whether she likes to have coffee or tea at certain times of the day, and what she likes in the beverage. Inquire whether snacking between meals is the norm. Routine and familiarity are cornerstones of habilitative care.

Consider what can happen if you don't know such details. When Rob's nursing-aide agency assigned him to be a live-in companion for Connie while her family spent a month vacationing, he thought the undertaking would be rather easy. Connie's family had described her as easygoing, affable, and pleasant. She rose early, spent most of the day in the garden, and retired by nine P.M. Although she was in the early stage of Alzheimer's, she had a profound loss of language skills. Otherwise, Connie was quiet and kept to herself.

Waking before Connie on their first morning together, Rob prepared a breakfast of bacon and eggs, which he set before her. He poured her a cup of coffee.

"Milk?" he asked. "Sugar?"

"Not." She shook her head, frowning, pushing the untouched plate away.

Rob pushed them back. "C'mon, Connie, you have to eat. I made these special for you."

Connie rose from the chair and went back upstairs to her room. Later she went out into the garden, and, unknown to the aide, drank water from the hose. Rob prepared a fresh pot of coffee for them and offered Connie a cup on the patio.

"Not, not, not," she said, her voice rising.

"What do you want? You haven't eaten anything. It's almost lunchtime. What should I make you for lunch? Do you want a salad? I'm going to make one for me. I'll make you one, too."

Connie returned to gardening. Rob prepared the salads, but again Connie did not eat (although she drank some more water from the hose).

Their interaction continued in that way, with Rob preparing meals and Connie refusing to eat and becoming angrier with each meal. Where was the sweet patient her family had described? Finally, sometime during the second week, Rob, at his wits' end, suggested that Connie go shopping with him.

"You pick out what you want. I don't care what it is. I will make it for you."

She seemed at first not to understand. Then, as they slowly ambled the aisles, she began touching familiar items. The first was tea bags. *Of course,* thought Rob. *Tea, she drinks tea, not coffee. No wonder she pushed the coffee away. Wouldn't you think the family would have told me?* He grabbed the box of tea bags and tossed them into the basket. Connie smiled. A new partnership was beginning.

Nothing could have been more important than for the family to tell Rob about Connie's likes and dislikes — where she liked to have her meals, what snacks she enjoyed, and what time meals were served. This kind of information not only keeps the patient scheduled and on familiar grounds, but helps to seal a positive relationship between the person with Alzheimer's and any temporary companion.

As the disease continues, the care partner needs to be on the alert for more serious issues concerning food. In the late stage, a person with Alzheimer's may have difficulties with chewing and swallowing, for instance. When such problems start to occur, the patient's physician or other health care provider should refer the person to a speech therapist. That specialist can give tips on the best feeding methods and types of food, such as soft, thick foods. These recommendations will maximize comfort for both the patient and the feeder.

Toileting

Thank you
for hanging a picture of a toilet
on the bathroom door.
Thank you
for not mentioning it.

Problems with toileting may arise in early stages or may not be a threat until the late stage. Over the past few decades, most clinicians who have worked with Alzheimer's patients have concurred that early in the disease, incontinence is not related to medical or physical causes so much as to environmental or other treatable conditions. Some people with Alzheimer's seem to think that it is safer to urinate outdoors than to try to find the appropriate place indoors. In many cases, the person once lived on a farm, was allowed to use the outdoors during the summer, or even had an outhouse as a young person. Being aware of the patient's background and social history enables family members and health care professionals to prepare for disconcerting situations such as inappropriate outdoor toileting.

The basic assessment for habilitative toileting includes learning whether the patient can find the bathroom and toilet, can indicate that she needs to use the toilet, and can undress quickly enough.

Marc awakened just after midnight, realizing that he had a strong urge to urinate. He rose from the bed he shared with Danielle, slipped into the sandals near his bedside, and went to the bathroom. Marc returned to bed and immediately fell back to sleep. Later Danielle reported that for three nights in a row, he walked over to the closet next to the bathroom, opened the closed door, and "peed all over my clothes."

Solving that problem was straightforward. Danielle stuck reflecting tape on the floor between Marc's side of the bed and the bathroom door. At night the tape acted as a one-inch-wide bright green pathway, guiding Marc to the bathroom at night. During the day the reflector tape did not show.

Also, Danielle used several inexpensive "touch" lamps in the bathroom to help Marc. (She had previously attempted to leave the bathroom light on many times, but frugal Marc would always shut it off before going to bed.) Danielle touched the lamp's plastic domes before retiring, so that a soft light emanated — just enough to offer a warm beacon to Marc as he approached, drawing his attention away from the closet and to the bathroom.

Danielle happily reported to a group of care partners that Marc had learned to use the bathroom, and she had successfully cleaned her clothes. (By the way, if urine odor is permeating a room of your home, the products offered to rid areas of the smell of cat urine work on human mistakes too.)

Danielle used some of the techniques I have found most helpful. Along with adjusting the environment to deal with the toileting issue, she replaced Marc's cardigans with pullovers to eliminate the struggle with buttoning, and she placed each day's medication in a small bright red plate at mealtime to draw his attention and aid his feeling of independence. She also greatly decreased his frustration when he was searching for a word by quickly saying it to him. These methods center around the patient's ability to find his way; attention span; depth, color, and contrast perception; fine motor skills; short-term memory; verbal abilities; and problems with medications or other illnesses.

To reduce visual problems, pick out a bright paint color that you can live with for a few years; turquoise, plum, terra cotta, and emerald green are great choices. Paint the bathroom walls a contrasting color to the toilet and sink, remembering that it's not likely that an interior-decorating magazine will be calling to photograph your décor. The white porcelain sink and toilet (and, perhaps, bathtub or shower) will be much more visible.

In many cases it is essential for the care partner to suggest to the person with short-term memory problems that it's time to make a trip to the bathroom. You can do this with habilitative language that does not imply that the patient needs to be reminded. You can say, "I think I'll scoot into the bathroom, Dad, why don't you go before me?" or "I'm going to use the upstairs bathroom, Mom. You can use this one over here. The one with these great blue walls." Many habilitative long-term-care programs offer two-hour toileting schedules; care partners guide residents to the bathroom while chatting about other matters. When they reach the destination, they say something like "I'll wait out here for you."

Because of short-term memory or attention-span problems, the person you're caring for may not equate the sensation of a full bladder with the need to find a toilet. Often, by the time the feeling is processed, he or she needs to get there speedily. Placing a stable commode at the patient's bedside may make nighttime toileting easier for both of you. And, as I mentioned earlier, have the patient wear elastic-waist slacks and skirts rather than tight outfits with buckles and buttons.

Also, place a disposable bed pad under the bottom sheet on the patient's side of the bed before nighttime incontinence becomes an issue. And if incontinence becomes a way of life, place sturdy plastic sheeting under the sheets, even if the patient is wearing diapers overnight. Eliminate fluids after evening meals if the patient is urinating during the night, and try to keep the bathroom door open and the light on. If a patient visits a friend or family member, mention her special toileting needs to the host.

Check with your physician if the patient you are caring for suddenly has problems controlling his bowels or bladder. You may find that a medication or illness is causing the problem. And if constipation becomes an issue, try adding stewed prunes, apricots, or other fibrous foods to the daily diet, and seek the help of a nutritionist if you need to. (A padded or elevated toilet seat can help make a long sitting more comfortable, and sometimes some soft music will help.) If the patient doesn't seem able to sit on the toilet long enough, give him a familiar object to stimulate interest in sitting. One or two photo albums, a magazine, dolls, or a busy apron may occupy the person long enough to accomplish the task.

And to help with patients' failing verbal abilities, when phrases such as "the women's room," "bathroom," or "lavatory" no longer have meaning, some habilitative facilities place pictures of toilets on bathroom doors. Plumbing-supply stores have books of appropriate bathroom photographs from which you can request one to hang at home.

Whatever techniques you try with a patient, do not treat early-stage incontinence by moving directly to geriatric diapers. Giving in to the lowest expectation will cause the patient to feel embarrassed, hostile, a failure. However, when the need for some incontinence measure is clear, you may want to begin by using women's sanitary pads as panty or underwear liners, which are easier to put on and remove than full diapers. Using pads along with a strict toileting schedule (every two hours), you may be able to defer serious incontinence for a while longer.

Finally, ignore accidents, and praise results. Your objective is to lessen the patient's embarrassment, shame, and apprehension. Habilitation offers the opportunity for long-term feelings of success — as well as dry pants.

Sleeping

In many cases sleeping problems are the final straw for the care partner; when sleeping becomes a major issue, the habilitator quite often admits defeat and starts seriously pursuing out-of-home care options.

Many people with progressive dementias sleep for only about

six hours at night. Those who take several naps during the day sleep even less after the sun goes down. You do not need to be a mathematician to figure out that if the person with Alzheimer's retires to bed at eight P.M. and receives a "good" night's sleep, she may be ready to start the day at two in the morning. The care partner may be just drifting off at that hour and is hardly ready to go back on duty to oversee waking activities. Add into that the care partner's worries that the patient may find hazardous items or areas or may leave the house.

The result is stress, tension, and frustration between patient and care partner, which can lead to outbursts. Those, in turn, add guilt to the care partner's emotional overload. No wonder that sleep deprivation of the worn-out care partner is a primary reason for seeking to place Alzheimer's patients in nursing homes.

Do not panic, assuming that all your nights as a care partner will be sleepless. Many people maintain the same sleep pattern they had before Alzheimer's disease became a part of their lives, or they develop a new, reasonable sleep pattern.

For some patients, however, night and day become twined together, and no care partner can unravel these mysterious threads of time. If changes in sleep habits occur, you should assess whether the disturbances are linked to physical, medical, or emotional events rather than to the disease process. The patient may be getting a cold or the flu, may be dehydrated or hungry and unable to relate her discomfort, may need to use the toilet, or may desire to open a window. Perhaps the designated bedtime doesn't work because she worked the night shift earlier in life.

When Charlotte came to the support group, she slumped into a chair. She had dark circles around her eyes. "Mother is up at all hours of the night. I have to get up so early to get the kids ready for school and get her ready for day care that I am exhausted by the time I get to work." Given the group's advice to find out if an unrelated problem existed, Charlotte took her mother to the doctor, who noted changes in the joints in her arthritic hands and knees and prescribed a medication to help with inflammation.

Soon afterward both Charlotte and her mother were sleeping through the night.

In another scenario, Elizabeth, who had Alzheimer's, suffered horrible nightmares until her husband discovered the cause quite by chance. One of their traditions as a couple had been watching the eleven o'clock news. Even after her disease had taken away her ability to comprehend a news story, Elizabeth sat each night staring at the sights and sounds flashing across the television screen. Then she would go to bed, only to awake screaming in the night. Only after their cable service was disrupted did Elizabeth's husband discover that the images on the screen of warfare, automobile accidents, and assorted acts of mayhem were causing his wife's nightmares. As soon as they stopped watching the news, Elizabeth began to sleep peacefully until dawn.

Whatever the reason for the patient's sleep problems, the care partner should establish a truly habilitative environment to protect the person at risk. You will be able to rest easy if you have carefully put away all dangerous household items, placed childproof locks on cabinets, and installed bells or traveler's locks on doors.

Other suggestions for creating a habilitative setting for sleep include singing or using a tape recorder to softly play a lullaby in the bedroom. Familiar, comforting tunes can induce sleep for older people, just as they do for babies.

And if the patient's sleep-wake cycle seems confused, try keeping her awake all through the day until bedtime. You may need to start gradually by keeping a record of the times when she naps during the day. Once you find the pattern, arrange to take a walk with her ten or fifteen minutes before she usually falls asleep during the day. Eventually, she will sleep longer during the night. Naps during the day often reflect boredom, as well; the patient may need some new task, chore, or hobby to keep busy with.

An evening stroll helps to relax both care partner and patient in preparation for a good night's rest. And don't underestimate the soothing effects of warm milk and back rubs. My mom paid her grandchildren to rub her feet with glycerin and rosewater. At ninety she still had beautiful tootsies and always slept like a baby.

A sleeping medication for the patient might become necessary to enable the care partner to get a good night's sleep. At home the medicine may be needed much sooner than it would be in a nursing home. If you go this route, recognize that many choices of sleeping medications exist, along with many controversies about the drugs. Of course, consult with your doctor or pharmacist, and tell them about the patient's body size, age, diagnosis, and any other medications he is taking.

Whatever you do, recognize that if the person you work with develops a sleeping problem, you must find support and relief of some sort. You might have a "family sleepover," letting several family members take turns being the "guard" during the night. Or have a home-health aide stay over occasionally. Both care partners and patients need a good night's sleep.

9

Tenet #4: Live in the Patient's World: Behavioral Changes

I can no longer
make apple strudel,
but I can chop pecans or roll the dough or peel the fruit.
I am here.
I've not yet gone.

NEVER QUESTION, chastise, or try to reason with the patient. Join him in his current "place" or time, no matter when or where that may be, and find joy with him there.

At a recent patient support group, I turned to a friendly woman next to me and said, "How wonderful to see you."

Puzzled, she looked at me for several seconds before saying, "Have we met before? You don't look at all familiar."

Even though she had attended the previous three meetings, I replied, taking her hand in mine, "It is always so nice to meet new friends." She smiled, noticeably relaxing as she grasped my hand. The accuracy of our interchange was unimportant; her self-esteem was all that mattered. Meanwhile, I had enhanced her day, and I felt buoyed as the care partner of the moment. I had entered her world, and it seemed like a nice place to be for a while.

A host of techniques can help you work appropriately with Alzheimer's patients as they encounter typical behavioral changes, such as not recognizing people and having difficulty making choices. To start with, when a patient's behavior seems to be changing, check out his basic physical comfort. Is he thirsty? Hungry? Does he have to go to the bathroom? Too hot or too cold? Overmedicated? Do hearing aids or eyeglasses need to be checked? Does he need to talk to someone about what is happening to him?

Remember that the person may not be able to communicate in words what seems to us to be simple information. Check often on her medical and physical well-being to ward off negative behavior before it has a chance to appear. If she is out of sorts, cranky, agitated, or aggressive, first determine whether she has some illness or physical discomfort that she may be unable to articulate — constipation, arthritic pain, sore throat, earache, headache, or bellyache. An impending illness or other physical ailment may be the cause of the distress. Have the patient's primary care physician check her for any medical problems before assuming her behavior is just another trial of Alzheimer's.

If you have to take a temperature, try to do it before a meal to ensure the most accurate reading. If the patient refuses to let you take her temperature, buy a second thermometer and take your own temperature at the same time, explaining that the doctor is checking everyone for flu.

How to Deal with Typical Behavioral Changes

The behaviors listed here roughly follow the order of the list in Chapter 3 of behavioral changes as the disease progresses.

Forgetting Appointments or Events

If a person in the early stage of Alzheimer's forgets an appointment, don't make her feel that she made a mistake; it's far better to make up an excuse or blame the incident on an intervening event: "It's just as well; the doctor was running late anyway."

Losing Track of Time

In the early stage, an Alzheimer's patient may forget that he just ate and, ten minutes after polishing off a sandwich, announce that he's hungry. Rather than saying "You just ate," distract him — "Oh, look, your favorite show is coming on" — or somehow modify his behavior: "You know, I'm still full from lunch. Let's have tea now, instead of dinner."

Repetitiveness

When the person with Alzheimer's repeatedly asks the same question ("What time is it?!"), keep in mind that she doesn't want the *question* answered; rather, she wants to articulate some feeling behind the question. What is her face saying? Try to find the meaning, the emotion, behind the query. The two most common questions that occur daily are "What time is it?" and "Where is my mother [or father]?" The question about time means that the patient is asking for something to occupy her time. The second question means that she is seeking comfort and reassurance.

Not Retaining Information or Memory of Events

When the person shows that he has forgotten some information or event, don't try to help him remember it. Simply change the subject and move on to a subject he is comfortable with. Or discuss the event from your own frame of reference. If, for instance, he has forgotten attending a recent wedding, you could say, "Oh, we had such a lovely time at the wedding. We saw your cousin John and ate chocolate wedding cake." Include the patient in the memory: "You and I danced until eleven o'clock." It doesn't really matter whether the details are accurate — some memories can use a bit of dressing up.

A patient in the early stage who is independent enough to do some things alone may still need some help remembering certain information. Peggy, for example, had trouble at the checkout line of a market. When told the bill, Peggy handed Lynn, the checkout person, a quarter and a cherry Life Saver and whispered, "How's that?" Knowing about Peggy's situation, Lynn was able to help her find the correct amount of money. The patient should be guided to establishments where personnel are acquainted with her needs and won't embarrass her.

Many chapters of the National Alzheimer's Association offer a small, wallet-sized "memory" card that a patient can carry. The card states, "I have a memory problem. Please be patient." Or a care partner can easily craft a similar card.

Not Recognizing People

If the person with Alzheimer's fails to recognize you as a friend or acquaintance, simply reintroduce yourself. You've preserved his self-esteem, and the conversation can continue smoothly.

Word-finding Difficulties

When the person with Alzheimer's is struggling to remember a word — either written or oral — simply say it to her if you know it. The more time that is wasted searching for the word, the more likely that the person will lose the thought altogether. Your goal is to make communication as smooth and easy as possible.

Difficulty Making Choices

Remember that you cannot reason with someone who has lost the ability to do so. Instead, limit any choice to two items: "Shrimp or steak?" "Black dress or red?" (The person will probably choose the second possibility, making the "last-word connection," as I mentioned in Chapter 7.)

Diminished Concentration

Keep a task going for a manageable length of time, bringing it to a close before the patient becomes exasperated. A care partner is generally able to tell when the person is getting bored or frustrated, signs that he will soon flare up or express unhappiness.

Accusatory Behavior

Since the patient has lost the ability to reason, agree immediately with her version of events or offer a very reasonable explanation for her concerns. To the accusation "You stole my special coat," the answer is "I forgot to tell you that I put it in storage for the summer," even if the coat was sold twenty years ago. For "The aide is stealing," the answer is "I'll talk to him. It won't happen again." (Of course, tell the aide about the false accusation and your habilitative response, so that he understands the need for this white lie and stays on your side.) Paranoid behavior is usually directed at the closest family member, and that person should remain in the patient's world throughout the discussion, no matter how bizarre the accusation.

Difficulty Separating Fact from Fiction

Since a patient cannot always be in our world, it becomes essential to monitor where she is in her interior world — and to join her there if necessary.

Todd and his wife, Lucy, were watching the presidential election convention on television. Lucy, in the middle stages of Alzheimer's, became increasingly restless. Todd turned off the TV to assess her obvious distress. Immediately Lucy breathed a great sigh of relief and said, "Oh, thank God. I didn't know how we were going to feed all those people." She had perceived all the conventioneers as being in her living room.

"I took care of that," Todd replied, smiling. "Now there's just the two of us. Let's eat. I'm so hungry."

Todd, practicing habilitation, did not chastise Lucy for her impossible scenario, nor did he try to reason with her or explain why these people could not be in their living room. He simply went into her world for the necessary moment to reassure her, then changed the subject and turned it into a pleasant experience.

Impaired Ability to Translate Thoughts into Actions
At first, this behavior may be difficult to figure out, since the only thing that is apparent is the person's frustration. If you notice that the patient is acting frustrated, it may be that he cannot perform the task at hand or cannot communicate what he would like to do. Distract the patient with another task, food, or a different situation.

Changes in Judgment
People in the late early stage of Alzheimer's have an impaired ability to make and remember judgment calls. Someone at this stage can reach out and touch a hot stove, burn himself, and ten minutes later reach out again to touch the same hot stove. He may have difficulty understanding the weather — going outside in winter, for example, without boots, hat, gloves, or coat.

Constantly monitor a patient for the ability to make and recall sound decisions. Try to make the environment interesting enough, simple enough, and safe enough to avoid problems before they start.

Diminishing Ability to Sequence Tasks
If the patient has difficulty brushing her teeth, put toothpaste on the toothbrush, place it on the counter, and leave the water running *before* she goes into the bathroom. If she wants to bake a cake, measure the ingredients ahead of time and put them on the counter. And don't call attention to what you have done.

Difficulty Writing and Understanding Written Language
Before writing difficulties become pronounced, try to take over any writing chores. Monitor the situation for frustration, and distract the patient if necessary.

When a patient no longer understands written words, don't speak about it or ask questions about what she is reading. You don't need to take away books and magazines — keep them around if she is used to them.

Getting Lost in Memories

If the person with Alzheimer's mistakes someone for a person from the past or thinks he is in a different place entirely, allow him the leisure and liberty to take you where he wants you to go.

Not all memories are pleasant ones, of course. If, for example, the patient starts crying because she sees a parent in the mirror, acknowledge the issue ("It's making you unhappy to see your mother right now, I understand"), distract the patient ("Here, have a cookie"), and remove the trigger of the unhappiness (get rid of the mirror). Happy or not, though, getting lost in memories may indicate that the patient needs to discuss the past — perhaps not at that moment, however.

Impaired Computation Abilities

When you notice that the patient is having trouble with simple math, you will have to be ready to take over or oversee any transactions that require an understanding of numbers. This includes balancing the checkbook, paying bills, making change, paying a cashier, leaving a tip, measuring for recipes, reading a thermometer, setting the oven timer, and many other such tasks that we do daily. Guide the patient or take over as inconspicuously as possible to allow him to maintain a sense of control for as long as possible.

Changes in Reaction Time

When the patient begins to take a long time to react to a situation, do not put him in a situation that will require quick reflexes, such as baby-sitting or driving. If he was once a great ball player, but now his slower reactions make playing outfield impossible, toss him a large rubber ball in a game of catch. Don't stop playing! Even though reaction time is slower, that does not mean the person with Alzheimer's must now be excluded. The caveat, of course, is safety.

Not Recognizing Objects
This occurs especially with dining implements (forks, spoons, knives), keys, and other small objects. Eliminate all items that the patient no longer recognizes, even eyeglasses, hearing aids, and dentures. Don't try explaining what the object is for; that results in a sense of failure as well as confusion and frustration.

Lack of Social Appropriateness
Social graces may disappear when self-control no longer exists. "You have big boobs," a patient once told me, her loss of inhibition and control allowing her to say whatever she saw as the truth — much as a youngster will often do. You will have to judge each social situation as it arises to decide whether the patient's lack of social appropriateness will be problematic. Dinner at a dear friend's home is quite different from cocktails with your boss. Remember above all else that it is the disease causing the behavior and not the patient's desire to be naughty or to embarrass you. There are no medications to curb the lack of social appropriateness, but this stage will pass as the disease progresses. And if you *really* want to know how your new hairdo looks — just ask him!

Frequent Emotional Changes
Sometimes the patient will experience a whirlwind of emotions — laughing one minute, weeping the next, then laughing again. Follow the patient's lead and go with her emotion; remember that it is real to her. And remember that these outbursts are generally short-lived.

Problems with Holidays
Holiday celebrations can be difficult for people with Alzheimer's because they can't perform as they used to, and they're aware of it.

So much is going on, and they don't feel as if they're part of the action. Try to convince a patient to help in whatever way he can. Making the family's traditional Thanksgiving apple strudel may no longer be possible, but perhaps he could help roll out the dough.

Formulate a specific plan of care for the holiday. Plan on having the person with Alzheimer's be with only one person at a time, to cut down on confusion and overstimulation. Ahead of time, assign different people to be with her at particular times. Someone should always be with the patient, without her knowing that this has been planned. Be sure to have a secondary plan as well. You may have to leave the event if the patient has an outburst, for example. In that case, who will accompany the person home? Is everybody ready to leave, if that's the best solution?

Not all situations, of course, can be anticipated and outlined here. When confronted with a new behavioral change, keep the following solutions in mind:

- Don't reason with someone who has lost the ability to do so.
- Distract the person with another task, situation, or thought, instead of dwelling on the problem.
- Follow the patient's logic or thought pattern, entering her sense of reality. Then gently lead her back to your world.
- Don't hesitate to use white lies to keep the situation manageable.
- Physically remove items that may cause problems.

Because habilitative techniques have not been widely used in the past, common behavioral changes have truly been challenging to well-intentioned care partners, both professional and family. The use of habilitation techniques will do much to help everyone feel more comfortable in dealing with these challenges.

Aggressive Behavior

I did not mean to strike you.
I was protecting myself
against insensitivity:
My-self defense.

Jeanne sat in her favorite spot facing the large bay window and the bird feeders she had hung so carefully so many years ago. She smiled as the chickadees landed and pecked away at their lunchtime snack. Carolyn, Jeanne's home-health aide, entered the room and, not wanting to break Jeanne's limited concentration, walked softly behind the chair. She leaned over and placed the lunchtime bowl of chicken noodle soup on the table. Jeanne picked up the bowl, stood, slowly turned toward Carolyn, and threw the warm liquid in her face.

"Get out of my house," she screamed. "Get out now! Right now, or I'll call the police!" Jeanne picked up a magazine lying nearby and threw it as well, then ran after her aide, yelling, "Go, go now, I'm calling the police!"

This kind of behavior is known as a "catastrophic reaction," an overreaction to a situation created, usually, by a care partner or by the environment. In the above scenario, the sudden appearance of the aide and the soup startled Jeanne, so she reacted to protect herself. The situation had confounded and therefore frightened her.

Carolyn did leave. She sat in her car for a few moments, wiped off her soup-spattered face, removed her sweater, and returned, this time to the back door. She knocked gently and, when Jeanne answered, Carolyn took a deep breath, smiled, and said, "Hello, I'm Carolyn. I've come to do some chores for you. Where do I begin?"

"Come on in," Jeanne said. "Would you like to have a cup of tea with me?"

Aggressive behavior such as Jeanne's is the greatest concern for many care partners and provides the most fodder for discussion at family support group meetings. Such behavior is upsetting and possibly terrifying, particularly for a frail, elderly care partner who has never before been confronted this way. Fortunately, because the behavior is usually the result of a care partner's action or of the environmental setup, it can be avoided. If Carolyn had approached Jeanne from the front and told her what she was doing, Jeanne would not have been frightened and felt it necessary to defend herself against something that she simply did not comprehend. Had the aide announced as she approached that she was bringing in the soup, then stated that the soup was "chicken noodle today," Jeanne would have been aware of Carolyn's presence and of the arriving soup. With that preparation, she would not have reacted catastrophically.

Aggressive or challenging behaviors can stem from many problems related to Alzheimer's disease. Paranoia, hallucinations, repetitive behaviors, continual anxiety, changing sexual desires, or illness may cause the patient to act out or overreact. Using the habilitation approach, care partners and others who deal with patients with progressive dementia can come up with different, successful game plans to deal with challenging behaviors. Each care partner's approach will depend on many factors, of course, including his past and current relationship with the patient, his personal coping skills, and the available support systems.

Whenever you have to deal with challenging behavior, remember to make eye contact, speak calmly and slowly, and break down your speech into simple, short statements. It takes an emotionally charged patient even more time than usual to process language.

Unresolved issues that existed between the care partner and the patient before the onset of Alzheimer's disease may add to the challenge of dealing with behavioral matters. The care partner may think the patient is purposefully being obstinate or unreasonable, but that is not usually the case. If you think that a trying situation relates to your past relationship with the patient, talk to your doctor or a psychotherapist, presenting a realistic picture of how you and she interacted before progressive dementia complicated the picture.

No matter how dismaying a patient's "acting out" in public is for you or your family, it is usually not so stressful for the patient. When you have to deal with a challenging behavior in public, first recognize that, by and large, the behavior results from the disease. "It is not the person, it is the disease" is a favorite verbal reminder among my support-group participants. Care partners sometimes repeat this slogan aloud three or four times while their loved one is doing something embarrassing in front of neighbors or at the grocery store.

Ways to Reduce Challenging Behavior

Perhaps the most useful habilitation tool for figuring out the cause of aggressive and challenging behaviors is the Alzheimer's disease behavior log, which can isolate an underlying problem before it becomes serious. If the thought of keeping track of difficult behaviors sounds overwhelming — you probably feel that you have hardly enough minutes to do what is called for now — remember that if discovering the cause of the aberrant behavior leads to tempering or eliminating it altogether, the investment in time may make the difference between a frustrating and a satisfying day. Recognizing that certain confrontations are inevitable will also help you endure the disease. Time spent in anger, frustration, tears, and remorse is time wasted.

Keeping a behavior log involves collecting information of several kinds: the time of day, the exact location of the behavior, and a thorough description of environmental elements such as odors, sights, and sounds. Keep a record of these factors for each specific behavior and, generally, within ten entries you will see a pattern emerge that makes the trigger obvious. In the log it is also useful to record others' reports of the same behavior. Occasionally, you will understand the pattern after only three or four entries. The behavior may be triggered by the time of day, rainy weather, a visit by a certain relative, or a specific television show. When you know what to look for, you can then plan to keep the patient occupied during the difficult time slot; pull the shades on a rainy day and watch a video, perhaps, or explain the dilemma to the relative and ask that person to stay away until the behavior passes, or shut off the TV.

Here is the way a behavior log might look for Chad, whose challenging behavior is to bang loudly on the door with his fist.

Time, day, and date	Where	Full environmental description
10:15 A.M., Thurs., Oct. 5	back door	Cold outside and in — fire in fireplace — lights on everywhere in house — shades open — wind blowing — coffee brewing
2:04 P.M., Sat., Oct. 14	cellar door	Neighbors in for tea — light snow beginning to fall — wind blowing — candles lit — shades closed — house warm
6 P.M., Wed., Oct. 25	front door	Dinner placed on dining room table — house warm and cheery despite windstorm and blowing snow — church bells ringing in the distance

After only three entries, you can see that the wind was blowing each time Chad banged on the door. Evidently the sound of the wind evoked an emotion in him. What that emotion was doesn't matter; this information allowed the care partner to try to thwart the behavior before it caused more distress. Turning on soft music to mask the sound of the wind could work nicely. Keeping Chad occupied in a part of the house where he is least likely to hear the wind howl would be another option.

Here's another behavior log, this time for Laurie's unexpected frantic pacing:

Time, day, and date	Where	Full environment description
3:03 P.M., Sun., April 13	throughout the downstairs	Laurie's favorite TV show playing — curtains open — dinner is in oven — we are waiting for company and for the kids to come from the movies — I'm setting the table
4:11 P.M., Tues., April 22	downstairs hallway	Music is on — gray day. I am peeling potatoes. Kitchen lights are on. Draperies are drawn. Kids are at baseball game.
3:45 P.M., Fri., May 1	living room to front door and back	Preparing meal early to be ready for going out this evening. Kids are helping. Beautiful spring day — many neighbors out raking and gardening. Windows open and draperies too.

No need to make more entries in this log. Laurie begins her frantic pacing each day in midafternoon. Checking to see what is happening elsewhere, we notice that family members are active at that time. Laurie is sundowning, exhibiting her challenging behavior as the day comes to an end. This once busy homemaker appears to be confounded by her uselessness. Her mind may be racing: "What should I be doing?" "Are the children home yet?" "Have I made dinner yet?" "I have so much to do but I don't know what it is." Whatever she's thinking, the antidote for her sundowning is to fill this time period with some pleasurable contribution to the family life or, at the least, with work that distracts her.

Afternoon would be the ideal time to have someone take Laurie for a walk or to interact with her on an individual basis, particularly if exercise can be involved to dissipate some of the energy that Laurie is expending through pacing. If the children are home, they could be called upon to engage their grandmother in "helping" them with homework or outside chores. Assisting in the kitchen with readying the meal or arranging the dining table also could occupy the time now spent pacing.

Some experts speak of Alzheimer's as a disease of behavior. I think of it as a disease of the emotions, however. By understanding, working with, and to some extent controlling the patient's emotions, it is possible to encourage behavior that is acceptable. This approach works much better than running away from the challenging behavior or medicating the patient heavily. Of course, at times every habilitator will want to separate herself from the person with Alzheimer's and go into a quiet room where she can throw pillows, swear uncontrollably, or cry. That is a human response when someone we have known as friend, mother, brother, or husband has taken on a different persona, has become someone we don't know.

The behavior log can be remarkably helpful. In just a few seconds, you can record what happens just before the emotional change. After studying several records in the log, you can often determine the trigger and eliminate it. The patient will feel more in control of his world and will not build up his levels of frustration, agitation, and aggression.

Triggers for Challenging Behavior

Now consider some common triggers that can result in challenging behaviors, and how care partners can deal with these situations.

Paranoia and Hallucinations

One night Irene heard her husband scream, followed by a loud crash. She rushed into his bedroom to find him waving his cane and beating the white shade, which now hung in shambles from his window. A shattered lamp lay on the floor.

"Get out of here, you lousy bum. Get out of here!" Keith roared as he swung the cane.

"He's gone," Irene said softly as she stepped closer. "I saw him running across the lawn." She waited for Keith to calm down. Then, after he had lowered the cane, she said, "Come sit here on the bed. You're all out of breath."

Keith sat beside her, still panting, but reassured. Five minutes later, he put his head on the pillow and let Irene swing his legs onto the bed and cover him with a quilt.

By reacting calmly and immediately becoming part of Keith's world, Irene turned his fury into reasonable peace. She quickly realized that the stimulus behind Keith's hallucinating and paranoia was the shadow from the neighbor's flag moving across the window shade. The next day Irene replaced the shade with a darker color and put up some new, heavy drapes that she could close at sundown and so eliminate Keith's hallucinations.

Irene was also smart not to remind Keith later of the incident, which could have made him feel chagrined about losing his abilities. Many people with Alzheimer's have paranoia and hallucinations at some time during the disease. A patient might say, for example, "I hear people talking about me." Or she may blame others for things she has done or something she cannot make sense out of, resulting in comments such as "You're stealing all my money" or "Where did you hide my keys?" The way to calm such a person is to address the underlying feelings of fear, anxiety, or sadness, and to find ways to change the environment to lessen these problems.

Continual Anxiety

A patient who appears anxious can also create challenging situations. The person may repeatedly think about his past duties: having to get ready for the office, prepare lunch for a spouse, or be home in time for a child's school bus. Thoughts such as these may add to the anxiety he already has about the disease. If he isn't occupied for a time, he may suddenly say, "I need to be going home now," and try to act on that idea.

As you do with repetitive statements, think about what the veiled words really mean, such as "I need to feel useful right now." Again, giving the patient a task she can do may help her feel useful and still able to function as she did in the past. Even if she can no longer set the table properly for Sunday dinner, she may be able to put the silverware or plates on the table. If the plates wind up in the wrong places, so what? Rearrange them when the patient isn't looking and praise her for her help. Challenging behavior becomes far less likely when the person with Alzheimer's feels that she is still a functioning part of the family.

If continual anxiety is not easily modified, however, a deeper problem may be involved. Contact your physician for appropriate tests and, perhaps, medication that can ease the patient's suffering.

Sexual Behavior
Other challenging behaviors may deal with sexuality. The person with Alzheimer's disease has the same drives and desires as the rest of us but may have problems describing or acting on his sexual urges and in determining where and with whom the actions are appropriate. The patient may, in fact, develop a much stronger sense of sexuality, or hypersexuality. Changes in the brain may cause him to lose control and inhibition, resulting in sexual behavior that is disturbingly different from anything he has done in the past.

In the early stages of Alzheimer's, when the person's outward appearance has not yet changed, frustration often results from the loss of ability to communicate feelings about intimacy and sex. The person may be further upset if a care partner with whom she has been intimate is now uncomfortable speaking about sexual matters. When the disease has disrupted sexual expression and communication, a couple may need outside help to assure both partners that intimacy and affection can continue at this time when they are needed most. Just as a doctor routinely checks a patient's blood pressure and cholesterol level, she should ask about his physical needs and behaviors. If the doctor does not make these inquiries of the Alzheimer's patient, don't feel shy about bringing up the matters. A medical specialist, such as a nurse practitioner, may be able to offer advice.

An early-stage patient, after listening to a racy story or comment, may be unable to process the humor and join in with others' laughter. He may feign understanding, but underneath the facade feel lost, and even withdraw from the social setting. A care partner needs to vigilantly protect the impaired individual in such a situation, perhaps by reassuring him that the joke was obscure.

Later in the disease, the patient may not recognize her partner at times, or she may express sexual interest in someone else. In such situations, the care partner needs to be extremely sensitive and patient to keep both the patient's dignity and his own intact while struggling to deal with the situation. (Many care partners have told colorful tales of donning a wig or flirting outrageously with the unsuspecting spouse before inviting the patient into bed. Sometimes habilitation requires a great sense of humor.)

And if the patient expresses sexual desire much more often than in the past, remember that sexuality is not limited to intercourse. Intimacy includes touch, loving words, and so much more. An act as simple as a back rub may dissipate some of the sexual feelings that so often build up in a life in which normal sexual expression is blocked. Sometimes nothing is as wonderful as a hand rub or a warm hug. If the person with Alzheimer's is obviously intent on intercourse, treat the gesture as you would have in the past. If the early-stage patient becomes overbearing in the frequency of demands for sex or in making unsuitable propositions, to the point that you feel uncomfortable with the advances, then talk honestly about the issues. If hypersexuality becomes a problem in the more advanced stages, then speak to your physician about medications that will help subdue sexual urges.

If you are not the patient's partner or spouse and find yourself fending off unwanted advances, firmly but gently explain that this behavior is not appropriate for you. If possible, distract the patient with some other activity.

In some cases, behavior that seems to result from hypersexuality may come from a completely different need. A man who appears to be masturbating may actually have to urinate but cannot express the need. Someone with progressive dementia who is stripping off her clothes may just be too warm or may need to go to the bathroom.

Sometimes the healthy partner no longer feels a sexual attraction to the patient. If this reaction causes a care partner to feel guilt, failure, anger, embarrassment, or sadness, he or she should try to talk with other people who are experiencing the same feelings. A support group, private counseling, or discussions with a trusted friend can help.

Depression

Some other causes of challenging behavior may require medical intervention. Be on the lookout for signs that the patient is depressed and is no longer able to express his feelings. Signs of depression include napping frequently throughout the day, sleeping poorly at night, and having a poor appetite. Depressed patients are in great need of counseling so they can articulate fears and concerns. They also need to see a doctor to determine if short-term medication can alleviate the anxiety or depression.

We cannot feel what the person with Alzheimer's is feeling. But we can all recall the frustration of trying to remember a word or a name ("It's on the tip of my tongue") or the frustration that arises when we misplace our car keys. Multiply those feelings by one hundred, and you'll have a glimpse into the emotional state of the Alzheimer's person when he or she is acting out. Then slowly count to three, and respond to the patient as you would want someone to respond to you.

10

Tenet #5:
Enrich the Patient's Life

I am seeking,
I am not lost.
I am forgetful,
I am not gone.

CREATE MOMENTS for success, eliminate possible moments of failure, and praise frequently and with sincerity. Attempt to find joy wherever possible.

While driving into Boston one day, I received a call saying that my meeting had been canceled. Delighted, I took the next exit off the Massachusetts Turnpike and began to calculate whether I could stop by to see a family in distress and still surprise my grandson at his softball game. Then I wondered whether, if I planned my time right, I could return six overdue telephone calls while I watched the energetic nine-year-olds run the bases. I'm pleased to say that I was able to accomplish everything on that list. But, more important, I was able to plan, improvise, figure out shortcuts, and make choices about the order of these items.

How different my reaction to the canceled meeting was from

that of a person with early-stage Alzheimer's. The interruption in schedule might well have overwhelmed him. He might not have been able to figure out how to spend the free time, having few skills with which to think through and design a new course of action. Early on in the disease, carrying out chores, tasks, sports, hobbies, and pastimes becomes much more difficult, and friends and family members who once shared activities become unavailable.

The patient's loneliness is often compounded by the withdrawal of friends. Years after my husband's death, some of my friends explained that they simply did not know how to behave with him or what to say, and the fear of doing or saying something hurtful kept them away. Although they realized that their response to his illness was selfish, they were unable to overcome their feelings of discomfort. But the patient needs familiar visitors, and the care partner certainly needs the change offered by conversation with others.

As a result of this isolation, patients spend much of their time in apparent idleness. Care partners often complain that the person with Alzheimer's "just sits around all day." But in fact, while he may appear to be doing nothing, he is trying to think through his situation; because he is not being productive, he feels unworthy, valueless, undeserving — a failure.

As I've mentioned repeatedly, the person with Alzheimer's needs to have a sense of being a part of the society she lives in. She not only requires enrichment in daily life, but she also needs to feel that she is doing something that enhances someone else's life, just as we all do. Despite having a terminal illness, the patient wants to be considered a productive, contributing human being.

To help the patient fulfill these needs, the care partner needs to initiate activities, to plan and organize with creativity, resourcefulness, and a great degree of patience. Above all, care partners need to think of ways to compensate for lost skills, recognizing that even the simplest activity involves a sequence of steps that depend on cognition, recent memory, a sense of cause and effect, and a long-enough attention span. More complex activities involve motor skills, verbal communication, problem-solving, and patience.

Here's how Wendy, a care partner in a support group, altered the way she tried to engage her mother in a social activity. She first moaned to the group about the disaster she felt she had come up against when she invited some "friends from my mom's bridge club in to play cards. What a fiasco. Her friend Kate kept having to play the cards for her. I couldn't wait for them all to go, and I'll never ever invite them in again!" Wendy's mother hadn't been upset. But, Wendy said sheepishly, "I was having a nervous breakdown. The TV was on — they all love Jerry Springer — somebody was mowing the lawn, and there must have been half a dozen neighborhood kids running around our yard. I was so afraid she was going to do something wrong."

Recognizing that it's important to help Alzheimer's patients engage in sociable activities, the support group encouraged Wendy to try again. This time she arranged for the function to take place in the familiar setting of her home. She made sure that the get-together consisted only of women whom her mother knew well and that there were no additional stimuli, such as small children nearby or a television or radio playing in the background. Since her mother could no longer play bridge, Wendy came up with a simpler event — an afternoon tea — to fill time and maintain companionship. To help anyone who felt timid about conversing with Wendy's mother, who was struggling with language, Wendy decided upon a topic — a vacation the women took together — to start the conversation.

Wendy did invite her mother's friends over again. She listened to her mother giggle in the other room with her girlfriends as they reminded one another of their glorious week by the sea in "the good old days." "Weren't we devils?" she heard her mother say. Later, several of the women told Wendy that her mother seemed to have far fewer speech problems than she had had when they came over for bridge and seemed much more like her "old self." The memories of the long-ago vacation were more vivid for her mother than the recent card game.

Wendy had learned that trying to get a patient to perform the way others can causes more harm than good. Care partners should be honest and let visitors know that revisiting happy times long past makes for the most fruitful exchange. Giving friends and relatives an opportunity to rise to the occasion will not only make them feel good about their visits but will enable the patient to feel valued and appreciated.

Enrichment also means involving the person in tasks or chores. An Alzheimer's patient will be interested in a task for only a short period, because of her reduced attention span and limited patience. Still, she may find repetitive activities quite gratifying — folding, raking, polishing, sorting, whipping batter, planting. During tasks the care partner should remember to keep the patient included in simple conversation, even if her verbal skills are diminishing. And the care partner can use this as a time to hone his "emotional listening" skills. Working on chores also affords wonderful opportunities for the care partner to offer praise and gratitude for help.

Enriching Exercises

Another way to enhance a patient's life is to work on the mental-enrichment activities developed by neuropsychologist Dr. Paul Raia. The goal of the activities is to help the patient hold on to existing memory skills by stimulating parts of the brain that have not yet been used.

Dr. Raia's theory stems from research findings that older people can develop neurotrophins, hormones found most frequently in infants and small children, which are involved in making new connections among brain cells. Preliminary research has demonstrated that performing the kinds of activities Dr. Raia has worked out can result in the formation of neurotrophins, which allow the brain cells of Alzheimer's patients to make new connections and pathways around the area affected by the disease.

The fifteen activities below — which Dr. Raia calls "mental floss" — focus on stimulating areas of the brain that will eventually be affected by Alzheimer's disease. When you try these exercises with a patient, introduce them by saying, "Here are some activities that may help you with your memory." If the patient refuses to do them, don't force the issue; perhaps you can introduce them at another time. Be sure to start slowly and try only a few activities in one day. And if at any time the patient seems to be getting frustrated, agitated, or upset, slow down or stop the activity. Focus only on the activities she enjoys, since you want her to succeed.

What's the Main Idea?

Materials needed: tape recorder/player or CD (compact disk) player; book or short story on tape or CD.

Activity: listen to a paragraph from a book on tape or CD, then stop the recording. Ask the patient to tell you the main thoughts in that paragraph. Repeat this process five times using five different paragraphs. This activity helps memory and listening.

Touch and Tell

Materials needed: an opaque bag; miscellaneous household objects, such as a sponge, screw, button, plate, and candle.

Activity: place objects in the bag without letting the person see what they are. Instruct him to reach inside the bag and, by touch, identify each object. Repeat the exercise four or five times. This activity helps memory, sensory perception, and communication skills.

Mealtime

Activity: have the patient eat a meal with her nondominant hand. The purpose of this exercise is to transfer information from one side of the brain to the other, to build up the nondominant side. For this and other potentially messy activities, be sure to cover the person with a garment protector (see the Products section of Further Resources, page 223).

What Time Is It?

Materials needed: a piece of paper with ten clock faces drawn on it. The faces should have numbers but no hour and minute hands.

Activity: say aloud a particular time, such as quarter past ten, and ask the person to draw the hands on the clock in the correct positions. This activity helps physical and computing skills and memory.

Stimulating the Senses

Materials needed: blindfold.

Activity: blindfold the person and have her walk slowly through the house. Monitor her to ensure that she cannot bump into or trip on anything. This activity allows the person to pay attention to senses other than sight.

Banging along with Bach

Materials needed: a recording of music by Johann Sebastian Bach

Activity: play a recording of Bach (or any musical piece with an easy, steady, beat — preferably a 4/4 rhythm — that the person enjoys), and ask the patient to clap the rhythm. This exercise helps the patient focus.

Which One Is Different?

Materials needed: three index cards with magazine or newspaper pictures pasted on them. Two cards should have images that are similar in some obvious way; the third card should have a different picture. (For example, you might use two images of a one-story house and one picture of a two-story house.)

Activity: present the three index cards. Ask which card is different and why. This makes the person pay attention to visual details, hold things in memory, and make decisions.

Making Items with Clay

Materials needed: modeling clay.

Activity: ask the patient to form shapes of familiar objects — a car, a house, or even a circle or square. Forming things with his hands helps fine-motor control, while also allowing him to enjoy the feeling of touch.

Reading by Tens

Materials needed: a magazine or book, paper, pencil.

Activity: ask the patient to read, either aloud or to herself, a long paragraph from an article or book and copy down every tenth word. This activity involves counting, reading, focusing, and holding attention.

Stimulating the Sense of Smell

Materials needed: three or four small bottles or vials with caps; cotton balls; aromatic scents such as vanilla flavoring, orange peel, cinnamon, wintergreen mints and peppermints, vinegar, lemon juice, and ginger.

Activity: insert a cotton ball into each bottle, adding a drop or two of aromatic scent or a sprinkle of orange peel, cinnamon, or ginger.

If using four bottles, have one aroma that matches one of the other three. If using three bottles, have one aroma that matches one of the other two. For example, put a drop of vanilla into two bottles and orange peel into a third; a wintergreen candy in two bottles, and a peppermint candy in a third; ginger in two bottles and cinnamon in the third.

Take the cap off one bottle and present it to the patient, asking her to smell the bottle. Present each bottle in turn until the patient can identify the two bottles with the same smell and the one different bottle. This activity stimulates memory as well as the sense of smell.

Counting Backward

Activity: ask the person to count backward from one hundred by threes. Then ask him to count back by sevens, eights, and so forth. This activity stimulates memory and sequencing.

The Carrots on the Hat Rack

Activity: go to a particular area of the home and decide on a stopping place. For example, go to the front door and choose the hat rack in the entranceway as the stopping place. Then find another stopping place — the couch in the living room, for example. The dining room table can be the third stop. Make sure the person with Alzheimer's can name the three stopping places.

Then give the patient a list of three items — the more absurd the better — and ask him to visually associate one of these items with the first stopping place, a second item with the next place, and so on. For example, on the hat rack, he could visualize a hanging bunch of carrots. (The visualization's absurdity gives him the best chance of remembering the stopping place.) Next, take him to the first stopping place and ask him to visualize what goes there — the bunch of carrots in this case. Do the same at the second and third stopping places. This activity forces the person to use mental imagery, which is processed in a different part of the brain from memory. The exercise can help compensate for lost memory.

Floor Plans

Materials needed: paper, pencil.

Activity: ask the patient to draw a floor plan of her home and label the various rooms. Then ask the patient hypothetical questions — for example, "Say you were in the living room. How would you get from there to the bathroom?" Ask her to draw the route with the pencil.

This exercise helps the patient with mental images and spatial relationships. This visual problem involves thinking abstractly and seeing how things are connected.

Fun with a Puzzle
Materials needed: jigsaw puzzle with about fifty pieces.
Activity: ask the person to put the puzzle together. This task involves visual images and abstractions, as well as memory and fine motor skills.

Proverbs
Materials needed: a book of proverbs or a list you have made of proverbs.
Activity: read aloud a proverb, such as "A bird in the hand is worth two in the bush" and ask the patient to explain what it means. This activity helps abstract thinking, as well as verbalization.

More Activities for Early-Stage Patients

My colleague Lois Pecora, the director of Alzheimer's services for the Salmon Family of Health Care Services in Massachusetts, and I have shared facilitating both an early-stage support group and a care partner support group for the past five years. Here are a few activities that we use in our groups and pass on to at-home habilitators.

- Read a newspaper advice column and ask the patient to suggest responses.
- Challenge the patient to list as many words as possible that can be made from a longer word, such as "megaphone."
- Pose questions that have no wrong answer, such as "What three books would you take for a week's vacation alone?" or "What is your favorite dessert?" These kinds of questions will most likely foster further discussion on the chosen topic.

- Describe news, sports, or fashion stories of interest and ask for comments about them.
- Ask questions that involve making choices. For example, "Would you rather go on a picnic or to a five-star restaurant?" The answers can be a gauge of the person's ability to make decisions. At some point in the disease, the patient will reply, "Wherever you want to go" — or, using the "last-word connection" (see page 81), come up with an answer that involves no choice on his part.
- Describe a situation in the news and ask how the patient might solve the problem — for example, a budget deficit or a crisis in another country. Make sure the person understands that his response is of interest to you.

These are the kinds of conversational and thinking activities that well-organized adult day care and assisted-living situations offer in a social setting. A patient's failed attempts at conversation are usually met with chuckles, a pat on the hand, and a sly comment from another patient, such as "I know how you feel."

As you carry out any activity — whether in a social setting or at home — notice the patient's emotional state during and after the experience. As Dr. Raia has said, if you see signs of frustration, agitation, or anger during the activity, slow down or stop what you're doing. Also recognize that anger or befuddlement afterward may be triggered by something other than the activity itself. Try to identify the trigger and eliminate the problem causing the unwanted conduct or attitude.

A Daily Routine

Enrichment activities should be carried out within a structured daily routine. The need for routine doesn't mean you should curtail activities, however. A day filled with scheduled activities is often the catalyst for a night of pleasant sleep. An ideal, busy, practical, but quite attainable day in the life of a care partner and patient might include activities along these lines.

Early Morning

- Set the breakfast table together, according to the patient's ability.
- Have a leisurely breakfast, perhaps with a discussion of news headlines or sports news.
- Do breakfast cleanup chores together, including putting food away and clearing, washing, and drying dishes.
- Complete the bathing and grooming routines. The care partner should guide the person to the bathroom, allow him to do as much as possible, and find ways to handle his possible boredom or frustration.

Midmorning

- Put on clothes. To cue for dressing appropriately, the care partner can remind an independent patient of the day's events. For instance, she might say, "It looks like good golf weather today." For the patient who needs more guidance, the care partner can put out clothes in the correct sequence, without the patient's being aware of it. If the patient needs assistance, the care partner can place the clothes in position at night, to head off a potential confrontation the next morning.
- Go for a walk or engage in some other outdoor exercise. If a companion or family member can accompany the patient, the care partner can do necessary chores during this time apart.
- Exercise indoors if outdoor physical activity is not possible. Many videos feature aerobics and stretching exercises for older people, and most senior centers have solid exercise programs. Many clinicians believe strongly that physical exercise

promotes the Alzheimer's patient's well-being while slowing the downhill course of the disease.

- Take a coffee or tea break. If the patient is losing too much weight, the care partner can introduce a nutritious snack at this time. If weight gain is the problem, the habilitator can offer a light snack that will fill the void a bit before lunch. (See the finger food suggestions in the Appendix, page 207.) A snack at this time can be a reward for tasks already completed, which also means another chance to offer praise.

Late Morning

- Relax together, perhaps by watching a video, looking at a photo album, or reminiscing about past experiences (particularly those that elicit humor). If the patient is interested, she can pursue a hobby or avocation by herself. (This also lets the care partner finish chores.) A leisurely manicure followed by a hand massage will calm both patient and care partner.
- Weather permitting, take a short drive to nowhere or walk to a favorite local store. Sometimes an outing relieves the person's feelings of confinement and breaks up the monotony of being at home for long periods of time. The patient also gets a little exercise before mealtime. The care partner should be acutely tuned in to the patient's behavior after returning home. If problems arise, it may be better to stay at home, where the patient feels safe.

Noon

- Work together on lunch preparation. The care partner should guard against the patient feeling a sense of frustration or failure if he cannot complete the assigned task. The care partner should keep the table setting as simple and uncluttered as possible, and offer praise for any help.
- Eat lunch. The care partner may find it convenient to offer

the largest meal at lunchtime, and that is better nutritionally for the patient than a large evening meal.

- Do lunch cleanup chores together. The patient may function best at this time of day. Chores offer opportunities to feel useful and successful.

Early Afternoon

- If the patient doesn't have a problem sleeping at night, she can nap for an hour or less.
- If she has difficulty sleeping at night, have her engage in some sedentary activities. If she is able, she may be pleased to play card games, word games, or puzzles, to read, watch an old movie, or work on hobbies or projects. (As the patient's skills decline, the chosen activity should become less difficult.)
- Exercise enjoyably by taking a long walk, engaging in a sport such as golfing, dancing, or gardening, or doing household tasks.

Late Afternoon

- Take a coffee or tea break. Try to include other people at this time. A close friend or relative may be able to spend some time with the patient, giving the care partner some respite. Many people may be pleased to be asked to spend time with the patient and to help the care partner.
- If practical, work together on dinner preparation and table setting. A person with progressive dementia tends to have more cognitive difficulties late in the day (sundowning). He may require a lot of attention, so meal preparation may have to take second place.

Evening

- If the patient needs to retire early, perform bedtime preparations — brushing teeth, washing up, taking a sponge bath, putting out tomorrow's clothes. (Often people with Alzheimer's feel more secure when they have finished these chores.) As in the morning, the care partner should guide the person to the bathroom and allow her to do as much as possible for herself.

- Prepare for sleep, including putting on nightclothes and slippers.
- Relax in various ways, perhaps by listening to music, watching television, playing cards, taking a walk (preferably before changing into pajamas), singing, even dancing around the living room. (Doing the same activity at about the same time each day establishes a routine of sorts and may lessen stress and anxiety. This may be particularly valuable for patients who experience occasional sundowning.)
- Go to bed. The care partner may soothe the patient by giving a back, hand, or temple massage. Reading a poem aloud, even if a care partner has never done this before, often helps a patient fall asleep. The cadence of a metered poem read in a soft voice is very soothing. (Shel Silverstein's humorous poetry provides a great beat and can bring out a smile.)
- Ensure that alarms are set, doors locked, lights on in the bathroom, and preparations finished for tomorrow to make the day less stressful.

You can alter this schedule as necessary, of course. For instance, in the early stage of Alzheimer's disease, television can play a significant role in filling leisure time. This is fine, provided that the care partner exercises a little judgment in finding shows that engage the patient's mind — such as sports, nature shows, documentaries, or comedies. As the disease progresses, however, television may be overstimulating. As in the case of the woman who had nightmares after watching the news, the impaired adult may not be able to separate what is happening on the screen from real events. Select appropriate material that is simple to follow, and perhaps has just one voice speaking at a time (PBS or Discovery Channel documentaries, for example). Videos are also a good choice. Look for travelogues, videos from family gatherings, musicals, old television shows like *I Love Lucy*, and any favorites of the patient.

Physical Activity

Physical activities provide benefits beyond increasing strength, flexibility, and cardiovascular health. Exercising together affords both companionship and opportunities to participate in sensory activity. While walking, for instance, the care partner can talk about various odors in the air, can compare the bark on different trees, touch leaves on bushes along the way, or listen to bird songs.

Household tasks, both indoors and out, can be energizing and strengthening and can provide the best opportunities for praise and positive feedback. Remember that in later stages of the disease, the person may need a demonstration to initiate a task. But once the patient begins the task, he is likely to continue doing it for a while. After the early stage of Alzheimer's, you should plan any activity for no more than a half-hour, but you may find that the person wants to engage in some activities for a long time. Always, the object is not to complete the task but to be enjoyably occupied doing it.

Offer repetitive physical tasks, such as raking, planting, weeding, or vacuuming in the morning, when a patient's energy tends to be at its peak. Later in the day, physically repetitive activities may help tire the patient in preparation for a nap or bedtime. Don't complain if the person does the job repeatedly; just thank her profusely for helping with chores.

For every activity, prepare the supplies in advance; you run the risk of problems if you keep the patient waiting while you gather the necessary implements. Also, do not ask if he or she "wants to do" something; either begin doing the task or simply state the time when you will begin.

Most important, whatever you and the patient do during the

day, be sure to time activities with his previous routine in mind. Routine underscores a patient's feelings of security, well-being, and orientation. While you will have to make some compromises, your objective is to structure the patient's day while providing necessary time for other people to carry out their routines. A hired care partner or companion should also stick with the established routine throughout the course of the disease. Following the same course of events each day may be as important as any activity.

Keep in mind that activities are whatever we engage in to keep busy; they are the opposite of sitting with nothing to do or not knowing how to do anything. Keep the patient busy to fill leisure time and feel connected to the world through activity. Although much is lost, much remains. Focus on what is left, not on what is gone. Plan for contingencies, prepare for the terrible times — but use the techniques of habilitation to celebrate what can still be celebrated.

Enriching Activities

Try to fill empty times with activities that are creative or helpful, emotionally or spiritually enriching, or that offer the patient physical or cognitive benefits. Many of the activities in this list provide multiple benefits, and many can be used in nursing homes and assisted-living facilities.

Music
• Listening to music
• Engaging in sing-alongs, particularly of well-known, older songs
• Playing rhythm instruments
• Dancing
• Watching videos of musicals (especially older ones)

Food Appreciation
• Smelling and tasting foods with strong odors that evoke memories
• Feeling dough, Jell-O, pasta, and other foodstuffs
• Decorating cakes or cupcakes

- Making a salad or fruit compote from a set of ingredients placed on the counter
- Mixing ingredients for making latkes
- Preparing and baking cookies, cakes, or homemade bread
- Making applesauce
- Canning fruits and vegetables

Crafts and Hobbies
- Making and looking at mobiles
- Looking at or making scrapbooks and photo albums
- Making family collages, perhaps with seasonal themes
- Working on holiday projects, such as making valentines
- Arranging flowers, either fresh, dried, or silk
- Stringing popcorn or cereal loops to hang out for the birds
- Stuffing pinecones with peanut butter and seeds and hanging them for birds
- Dyeing Easter eggs

Spiritual, Inspirational, and Touch-based Activities
- Stringing beads for others
- Sewing, quilting, or making artwork for others
- Attending religious services
- Bird watching
- Spending time with pets in the home, visiting pets in other homes, or inviting someone with a calm pet to visit
- Cutting theme pictures out of magazines
- Sitting in the sun
- Walking on the beach
- Holding hands
- Receiving a massage
- Brushing hair
- Watching fish in a fish tank. The glass of the tank isn't dangerous, and the benefits of watching the fish far outweigh the grief of losing some. Even if the grieving period seems overly extended, it's all right for an Alzheimer's patient to feel grief.

Games
- Participating in trivia games, focusing on the eras the patient know best
- Playing "Finish the Pair," in which the patient tries to figure out the second item in a pair such as "Lucy and ____."
- Playing "Complete the Song Title," in which the patient tries to figure out the missing item in a song such as "You Are My ____."
- Piecing together jigsaw puzzles

- Answering "if" questions, such as "If ____ happened, what would you do?"
- Playing Pictionary — drawing a picture to explain the title of a television show, book, or movie
- Playing checkers, Chinese checkers, dominoes, or a children's form of an adult game such as Scrabble
- Playing simple card games, such as Old Maid or War

Outings*
- Spending time away with family or friends
- Collecting colored leaves
- Collecting beach glass or shells
- Building a snowman
- Attending social gatherings, as long as they are not overstimulating
- Going to cultural functions, such as dance performances or art exhibits
- Going to a library
- Shopping
- Taking historical bus tours through a city
- Traveling to a pick-your-own fruit farm
- Going to a nearby zoo
- Flying a kite

Activities to Stimulate Skills Affected by Alzheimer's

Verbal and Visual Skills
- Watching and discussing videos of old movies and television shows
- Discussing former occupations, service in the armed forces or other organizations, and past events, such as a first job, apartment, paycheck, or date
- Watching a children's performance or reading to children
- Being asked for advice about something the care partner is working on
- Listening to newspaper or magazine articles being read aloud
- Talking about great inventions and significant historical events
- Visiting or inviting in someone who has an infant
- Matching laundered socks

*After taking a patient in a nursing home or other facility on an outing, check with a staff member an hour or so after you return. If you find out that the patient became agitated after you left, suggest that in the future the staff have something ready for him to do upon his return. You may want to plan your outing to end just before a scheduled activity and have a staff member lead the patient into the activity as you depart.

- Looking at art books
- Writing a letter together

Motor Skills
- Sorting playing cards
- Tossing a ball
- Planting seeds outdoors or in pots indoors
- Clipping coupons
- Shelling nuts or peas
- Sorting buttons or screws
- Tossing bean bags, balloons, or a Frisbee
- Sorting playing cards by color, suit, or number
- Winding yarn
- Cutting seasonal or other thematic pictures out of magazines
- Polishing metal objects, such as brass doorknobs or candlesticks
- Helping to make a jack o' lantern
- Playing with children's clay (for patients with late-stage Alzheimer's)

PART THREE

Beyond
Habilitation

· 11 ·

Caring for the Care Partner

Applause does not always come easily.
You must be a winner
of both Scrabble and life games.
It is not always enough just to know
that lessons learned in apple orchards
may be lost on concrete streets.

Don't let care partnering take all the energy out of you. Consider Garrett, who rose from his bed at midnight, went down the front stairs, stopped at the front door, and jiggled the knob. He went to the back door and repeated the action, then he went back into bed. At one forty-five, he went back downstairs, rattled the front door and the back door, then walked around the house. Garrett headed back upstairs once more, put on yesterday's trousers over his pajamas, then padded, barefoot, back down to the kitchen door and out into the yard. He picked up the ax that lay beside the woodpile and, in the moonlight, began to chop.

Around four A.M., Garrett came back inside, barely noticing his wife, MJ, who was sitting on the stairs. They both sat down in the large recliner, as they had so many times before, and fell asleep.

Garrett did not have Alzheimer's disease; MJ did. Garrett was simply burning out from the stress of giving care around the clock. Many times he had gone without sleep, trying to be alert to any need MJ might have. Without adequate sleep, care partners cannot maintain their emotional stamina. As discussed in Chapter 8, sleep alterations are common in a person with progressive dementia; she may sleep less or nap at various times through the day and wake in the night just when the care partner is finally drifting off, hardly ready to oversee her nocturnal activities. Add into that the care partner's worries that the patient may find something hazardous around the house or even leave the house.

The result, for both the patient and the care partner, is stress, tension, and frustration, which can lead to outbursts. Those stresses, in turn, add guilt to the rest of the emotional overload. No wonder that sleep deprivation is a primary reason that worn-out care partners seek to place Alzheimer's patients in nursing homes.

Care for the care partner is mandatory. While every habilitator has heard this time and time again, it bears repeating. The patient's care will be nonexistent, or very problematic, if the care partner's physical or emotional health is challenged beyond repair.

Keep in mind a sobering statistic: 30 percent of all care partners die before the people they're caring for do. If the care partner is no longer there, all of the promises spoken ("Of course I won't let you go into a nursing home"), all of the sacrifices made ("It's okay, I'll eat/sleep/relax later") are for nothing.

You must learn to recognize your limitations and acknowledge your needs. Even the most effective care partner has, at times, been exhausted, resentful, and discouraged. You can't provide for the patient if your physical or emotional health is shaky. You should see your primary-care physician or a psychological therapist right away if you suddenly find yourself having some of the following symptoms:

- Mood swings
- Unusual irritability
- Inability to fall asleep
- Inability to stay asleep
- Difficulty concentrating
- Digestive problems
- Unfamiliar aches and pains
- Increased desire for or use of drugs or alcohol
- Sense of failure or hopelessness
- Frequent bouts of crying, fearfulness, sadness
- Lack of interest in normal activities or family

As we often hear, getting enough exercise, nutrition, sleep, and time off can help guard against undue stress. The trick, of course, is not to wait until you feel frazzled to begin the regime but to exercise, eat healthily, and sleep properly all the time, so that when the difficult times arise you can handle them as well as possible.

The demands on the habilitator often push exercise, for example, to the bottom of the priority list. Keep in mind that Alzheimer's patients who exercise appear to have less need for medications (for heart problems, blood pressure, arthritis, and so on), which is a compelling argument to find ways for both the patient and care partner to include an exercise program in the daily regime. Exercising together can mean sharing a walk, a bike ride, a swim, or a game of tennis. These times can also afford a chance to hold hands, reminisce, and find pleasure, and perhaps even joy, together. And while finding the time and energy to prepare nutritious meals may seem as arduous a task as painting the house, placing nourishing snacks in strategic locations, not buying high-sugar snacks, and eating an abundance of fruits and vegetables can help a great deal. Finally, if nighttime sleep is elusive, make time for an afternoon nap (or at least a moment to sit back with your feet raised) when the person with Alzheimer's is napping.

One more necessity is to find some time to relax. You need free time, however you find help. You must commit beforehand to taking time for yourself on a regular schedule, or you won't follow through on your plan. And that won't be good for either you or your partner. Within reason, don't let anything stop you from having your chosen time off. Maintaining a social life and participating in activities outside of caring for a patient with dementia helps to release some of the negative emotion that may be building — with or without your awareness.

You also need to create a calm atmosphere in some part of your home. Surround yourself with items that induce repose, perhaps by evoking memories of restful times and idyllic places. For instance, an herb garden with odors such as rosemary or basil may help. Potted plants, a goldfish bowl, a bird cage, landscape paintings or photographs of favorite scenes placed on walls, or colored stones or glass marbles in a bowl of water or a basket may take you to nostalgic places. Try a water garden, a basket of pinecones or sage, an arrangement of branches, or a bouquet of fresh flowers.

I have come up with an acronym to help remind you of your own daily needs: COPE.

C — Communicate, not only with the patient but also with the doctor, other helpers, and supporters. Let them know how *you* are feeling, not just how the patient is doing. Speak up. Mention your level of fatigue or feelings of burnout.

O — Organize and simplify the details of your own life and the patient's life. Organize drawers, closets, attic, and cellar, throwing away anything that's no longer needed. Go through old documents and organize those that have to be kept — discard the others. Get others to help you do this work. Simplify the house slowly — one room a week or a month until it is done. Place bills to be paid in an expandable file or set up another system that works for you. Being organized means you will have more time to spend being a habilitator.

P — Prioritize your time. What needs to happen next? Can some matters be done at another time? Make a timeline of how you need to proceed and include legal and financial matters, visits to long-term-care facilities, and appointments to find appropriate doctors. A regularly reviewed plan of care will prove helpful here.

E — Energize your body and your brain. Along with physical exercise, do crossword or jigsaw puzzles and listen to music and read alone or with the patient. Find time to use a computer or practice the piano.

If you don't see how you can possibly create time for yourself, give yourself permission to ask one or more people to help you. Friends and family members may be able to help, but so may the teenager next door (see Chapter 12 for an in-depth discussion of other people in the home). Use delivery services for groceries, meals, and other necessities to the extent that your geographic location and budget allow. You may want to invest in hiring a housekeeper, home-health aide, or visiting nurse.

You must wholeheartedly commit to taking time for yourself on a regular schedule; the benefits for both you and the person with Alzheimer's won't happen unless you do so. Decide in advance how much time you truly need each day, week, or month and incorporate that time into your plan of care. Will the patient be napping? Will he definitely be in bed for the night? Will you need someone to look in on him while you are away from the house?

Here are some suggestions for scheduling time for yourself:

- Twenty minutes every day for six months (then revise if necessary). Soak your feet, sit outside alone and listen to the birds, walk the dog, read a magazine in the park, talk on the telephone with a friend — this is twenty minutes at the same time every day just for you.
- Two hours every other week for three months (then revise if necessary). See a movie with a friend, have lunch with a

buddy, take a trip to the library, the hairdresser, or the bar-bershop, treat yourself to a bubble bath with scented candles, work out at the gym, have a massage, go on a bird walk, or work on a hobby.

• Four hours once a month. Play golf, go the museum, go to a spa and have "the works," have dinner with friends, go to the symphony, play bridge, mahjong, or poker.

Whole shelves of bookstores are devoted to various ways to re-duce stress and find relaxation, so I will not treat this subject in depth. The suggestions that follow are merely a few that I've seen work wonders in my own practice.

Specific relaxation techniques can ameliorate stressful situa-tions. Many medical centers have stress-reduction clinics that can help you learn methods that enable you to calm down and cope; for these, check out the clinics in your area.

One technique that I use with both patients and care partners, which works almost anywhere (in the car, the shower, around the home, on a walk) is a simple breathing exercise: Close your eyes. Take a deep breath through your nose, and exhale through your mouth. Repeat ten to twelve times.

Another technique is to sit down, relax your muscles, and vi-sualize the place where you feel the most relaxed. Try to push every other thought away, focusing only on that picture, letting it swallow up all of the tedium and difficulties in your daily life. A third technique is to focus on your toes, trying to relax them as much as possible; then focus on your feet, then ankles, calves, and so forth, until you work your way up to your head, making sure to relax your jaw muscles and the muscles around your eyes.

A Caution about Friends and Family

Some friends and family members may do more harm than good for you. One trait I see frequently is what I call the "Gee, He Looks Good to Me Syndrome." Friends and relatives often see what they want to see and don't understand how hard your situation is. A care partner once told me about a woman named Margaret, who said, as she left after a half-hour visit with her cousin, who had Alzheimer's, "He seems fine." But Margaret had not given her cousin a chance to talk, and he looked "fine" because the care partner had dressed him for the third time twenty minutes before the visit. At the end of such a visit, the visitor may turn to the care partner and essentially ask, "What's *your* problem [with the patient]?"

This situation often develops when a parent gets Alzheimer's and one adult child becomes the primary care partner. The other siblings are too busy or too far away; when they're finally forced to see the situation for what it is, they commonly say, "I don't know how you did it this long." Then they may become useful helpers. There's little that you can do about such misperceptions until the other person has the opportunity to walk in your shoes. Perhaps the person with Alzheimer's can stay with the relative for a few days, or the relative can stay with the patient while you're away "on business," if an excuse is needed.

In many cases, however, denial is the only way that people deal with Alzheimer's. In such situations, it's best to have the visitor visit as infrequently as possible.

You may have to be especially careful with family members with whom you or the patient has had difficult experiences in the past. Families for many reasons — particularly out of guilt — do not always acknowledge the good job the primary care partner is doing. It is a waste of time to hope that a relative's personality will change during this period. At some point you just may have to say, "You don't seem to understand, and your calling me [or visiting us] disrupts me and [the patient]. Please leave us alone."

Or the primary care partner may find himself barraged with supposedly helpful advice from someone who just wants to provide the advice, not the help. Listen if you choose; use the advice if you wish; but remember that you can say, "If you're not going to be here to help me, please don't make suggestions that I can't possibly do or handle." Use your energy to find solid support elsewhere rather than expending it on friends and relatives who aren't helpful.

Family meetings should always be encouraged, however, whether or not the family members get along. In therapy sessions with me, families often discuss issues they've had with the patient that have been under the surface all their lives. The only thing that has changed is that one member of the family has Alzheimer's, but the family dynamics remain the same. In such a situation, the crisis of dealing with the disease can actually be an opportunity to remedy long-standing negative family dynamics. But don't expect personalities to change just because a parent or other family member has Alzheimer's disease. Again: use the energy elsewhere. Accept pats on the back from anyone who gives them, and know that they are well deserved.

Support Groups

Once you recognize the importance of caring for yourself, you should seek a support group of other care partners. You need reassurance and validation; feeling the support of people in the same situation is a great beginning. A telephone call to the office of the local chapter of the National Alzheimer's Association should provide help in finding a nearby support group where you can share emotions, problems, and remedies with fellow care partners. Hospitals, nursing homes, assisted-living facilities, places of worship, libraries, councils on aging, and similar agencies host support groups that are generally open to anyone in the community. If at all possible, shop around and sit in on a few groups. Of course, not everybody can do this; some care partners may have to travel fifty miles to the nearest group.

Alzheimer's support groups offer families and friends an opportunity to focus on ways to care for the patient, skills to hone, humor to help you through the hard times, and education about the disease. Members find that they are not alone and have a forum to discuss ideas and concerns, to share hopes and even positive aspects of the disease. Giving others helpful feedback and offering compassion are steppingstones to your own self-care. This support system will replenish your energy as you gain the desire to smile through tomorrow.

A support group may also be able to provide clinical information about new medications and practical suggestions on how to influence a patient to stop driving, for example. Members may be energized to learn about organized advocacy or new strategies to help children deal with an afflicted parent. Remember that members steer the group meetings, so you can give to or take from your group as much as you need.

Generally, support groups are either closed or open-ended. Closed support groups run for a certain length of time (often eight to twelve weeks), with a group of people who have signed up. At the end of the specified time, the group disbands. These sessions are usually educational in nature, set up strictly for informational purposes. Open-ended support groups, on the other hand, meet year-round, through holidays and vacations, with no end date. New members may come into the group at any time. The facilitator of the group may be a care partner or a professional from a local assisted-living center or a nursing home.

Whether closed or open-ended, support groups can come in a variety of flavors. The most common are these:

- Early-stage support groups for caregivers (this may be the most common type)
- Groups for caregivers of mentally retarded adults with Alzheimer's (all people with Down's syndrome, for example, will develop Alzheimer's)
- Early-onset groups, for patients under sixty-five at the time of diagnosis
- Foreign/cultural support groups
- Men-only groups

• Groups for children of parents or grandparents with Alzheimer's

You may also want to look into early-stage patient support groups, which are for patients only. Such groups can be beneficial to the patient, who often feels able to communicate in this setting: instead of relying on wordless pleas for understanding, she finds others who can help her find lost words. Many family members who thought that a patient was unable to talk about her feelings have been surprised to discover that in a safe forum, with others bearing the same diagnosis, she could be remarkably insightful and articulate about these emotions.

The ideal is to find an early-stage patient support group and an early-stage caregiver support group that meet at the same time in one building but in different rooms. An option I find less effective is a single support group for both care partners and patients — often called an early-stage patient/caregiver support group. This option often doesn't allow either person to articulate her feelings freely.

Remember that support groups can go a long way toward reducing both emotional and practical stress. One of the best aspects is the opportunity for share-care (see Chapter 12), in which care partners in the support group take turns watching over several people with Alzheimer's — allowing the other care partners to have some personal time, with the knowledge that a trusted person is supervising the patient.

Caring at a Distance

You will also encounter stress if you are caring for a family member or close friend who lives elsewhere. Even if you are a long-distance care partner, you will still feel a loss of freedom, and you may well face anger, fear, and fatigue repeatedly. You might receive repeated telephone calls from another time zone — perhaps thirteen times a day or more. Or the manager of the apartment building where the patient has lived for the past six years might call you to report bizarre nightly behavior, wanting to know what you are going to do about the problem — and when.

To reduce your stress over the long run, begin as early as possible to keep a notebook about the faraway afflicted person's changes in mood, skills, behavior, cognition, and activities of daily living each time you visit. If the patient has some help, speak with the helpers before, during, and after each of your visits. Discuss the situation with the council on aging in the town where the afflicted person lives — perhaps you can arrange to have a case manager stop by and assess the situation. To get another opinion about the patient, contact as many people who know him as possible — neighbors, other family members, clergy. Determine whether the symptoms they mention are just signs of old age or indications of something more serious.

If you suspect that the person has Alzheimer's or some form of dementia, you may have to visit her and become an unpopular person for a while — especially if she is opposed to going to a doctor or getting a workup. You'll have to decide to take action, even if she will dislike you for it or do nothing, taking the chance that something terrible will happen that you'll have to live with for the rest of your life.

If you decide that an unwilling patient must see a doctor, you can take some steps to make the appointment more pleasant. Set up the appointment allegedly for yourself, and get the person to accompany you. Have an assessment done on him during that time. Or find a geriatrician who will come to the house — this is becoming a popular service. Your local chapter of the Alzheimer's Association will be able to recommend someone.

In most cases the person with Alzheimer's will have no helpers initially, so safety will become your primary concern. Touch bases with the Alzheimer's Association in the area and explain that you are a long-distance care partner, and you need to ensure the person's safety. Also, tap into the formal support network, which includes adult day care, home health care, the local Visiting Nurses

Association (VNA), Meals on Wheels, and any other supports that the Alzheimer's Association recommends. Frequently, the network includes sources of community help; ask for whatever help you think will be needed in the future. If your decision to bring helpers into the home meets with consternation on the part of the patient, point out that the aide's presence will ease your mind.

When you visit the patient, be sure to spend at least three or four days. Visit her friends, neighbors, primary-care physician, house of worship, closest hospital, and the council on aging. That will help you find out who and what services are available. Then, if a problem arises when you cannot make a quick trip to see the person, these contacts may be able to help out and perhaps even network with one another.

Set up interviews with medical doctors, home health care agencies, case management programs, and assisted-living centers and nursing homes. Take the time to visit them in person, using the assessment tools provided in Chapters 12 and 13. I have received many calls throughout the years from long-distance care partners in great distress after a hired helper has been brought into the home without an interview. Don't let this happen to you; visiting the various organizations and institutions will let you be prepared. (If you need to choose, say, a neurologist or a nursing home, narrow your choices to two in case one is booked when you need it the most.)

If you visit your loved one only at infrequent intervals, be prepared for changes wrought by the disease. Education about the disease process is a must. If you cannot attend a support group in your region, then get information from the library or the Alzheimer's Association on the manifestations of the disease and what to expect as it progresses (and see Chapter 3).

If you feel that the patient might be better off living near you, weigh all the possible alternatives before making the move. Consider whether the patient will have as many visitors and whether the care will be better. Do you want to visit her more often, and in a closer location? Would you like to take a greater part in her care? Are you considering the move to assuage your feelings of guilt? Will the move unsettle her and perhaps create new way-finding problems? Do the emotional positives outweigh the material negatives?

Maybe a move will help both you and the patient. Then again, the patient may see a potential move as an attempt to interfere with her life. Past history plays a major role in a patient whose long-term memories have become the bulk of today's thoughts. Trying to make up for negative past interactions by bringing your mother, say, to live with or near you at the end of her life may not buy you the solace you require. Your current relationships may have to take precedence over a relative living far away. Accept this situation with as little guilt as possible. Professional care partners who have learned the appropriate ways to interact with cognitively impaired adults can make the patient's life as good as possible. Often this arrangement frees the afflicted person from the stress of family history and the burden of having to perform well enough to hide the illness. An appropriate care partner will generally accept the person the way she is now. As she progresses through the disease, she will grow to love the care partner.

Be sure to show your appreciation to any far-away care partners. Call them often and offer praise and support. Send tokens of your appreciation and remember their birthdays. Whether friend, neighbor, or professional, they are helping you. And remember that every human being is unique and brings individual skills to the care-partnering experience. Don't compare your abilities with those of another care partner; we all have different resources — in terms of finances, family, personality, previous history, and more — to draw from. Don't be afraid to say aloud several times a day, "Not every marriage was made in heaven" or "Not every family relationship is okay."

Many years ago, I was at my grandmother's house after she died, going through her belongings. I came across an ancient faded box stuck in a corner. Opening it gingerly, I found a magnificent velvet hat adorned with tiny peach-colored rosebuds so perfect that I leaned down to sniff them, sure they must be real. A yellowed price tag still dangled from the brim.

"Why didn't Grandmother wear this beautiful hat?" I asked my grandfather.

He held the hat gently, the soft velvet a contrast to his rough flesh. "She was saving it, honey," he told me. "She was saving it for a special occasion."

Any moment can be a special occasion. A care partner needs to reduce the stresses in his life so that he — and the person he is caring for — can feel the special quality of their time together. As a care partner, try to *savor* more moments and *endure* fewer.

· 12 ·

Receiving Home Care

I am not running fast enough
to keep away
that furtive shadow chasing me.
Next I'll breathless stop
to find that same shadow
is all that's left of me.

Shay McGraney, seventy-nine years old, was in the final stage of Alzheimer's. She spent her time in bed or looking out the window at her younger brother Edward's house in coastal Oregon. Edward had pasted a poster of the Irish countryside on the ceiling above her bed. A cassette player issued soft Irish music as a part-time home-health aide tucked in the rumpled blankets. Shay smiled.

She no longer used words to express thoughts. But Edward and the aide recognized the subtle facial movements that indicated when she was cold or thirsty, and they responded to those needs. Edward understood that Shay no longer knew how he was related to her. But he knew that she felt loved.

Home care is rarely as idyllic as that. But it can be the ideal situation for both patient and care partner — if, and only if, both are comfortable with the arrangement, if the past history between the two has been positive, and if the care partner wants to perform the care out of love, not guilt. If all those pieces are in place, home care can be the best choice because it enables the patient to remain oriented to the world as much as possible and is the easiest setting for implementing habilitative methods.

All care partners need to learn about what formal and informal support systems are available. Keep in mind that as the disease progresses, the person with Alzheimer's will require additional or different types of assistance; what is appropriate today, when the person is living alone in her own home, will be inappropriate tomorrow, when she is no longer able to take care of personal needs.

Here are the resources most commonly available, which are discussed in this chapter:

- Home care by one or more habilitators: Even if you are the primary care partner in your own home or the patient's home, you may also enlist other people to help with the care.
- Home health care agencies: These agencies provide personnel, including aides and housekeepers, for a variety of tasks in the home.
- Case management programs: A social worker from this program will set up and manage a plan of care.
- Adult day health centers: These centers offer enrichment activities to early- and middle-stage Alzheimer's patients. They have trained staff and may also have a trained nurse on the premises.
- Adult day care centers: Day care centers offer enrichment activities for all adults with medical problems; they may not have trained staff or an available nurse.

Home Care by a Habilitator

Home care is often the first and best choice for both patient and care partner. The surroundings are familiar and can be modified as the patient's condition changes.

At home you can monitor visitors — people both known and unknown to the person with Alzheimer's — more easily, so social situations are often more pleasant and more predictable. Routine activities of daily life will be less challenging for the patient because household objects are where they're "supposed" to be; odors are familiar; and the caregiver remains constant, without any surprising changes of staff or personnel. The person's hobbies, tools, and interests continue to surround him; leisure activities can continue relatively unchanged, so it is easier to fill up the day. Personal memorabilia provide opportunities for reflection and conversation. Being surrounded with much-loved objects in a long-known setting is one of the basic ways to keep an Alzheimer's patient in touch with the world: if the world is familiar, the patient feels more secure.

Home care is the most common solution to Alzheimer's. According to the 2001 National Public Policy Program of the National Alzheimer's Association, 70 percent of people with Alzheimer's disease live at home, with approximately three fourths of home care provided by family and friends.

Before making the decision to become the primary care partner for a patient, assess the level of involvement that other people can assume. If the person with Alzheimer's lives alone, you may want to have a delivery service bring in groceries or other hard-to-carry items. If the person with Alzheimer's is living with the care partner, you may want to investigate local Meals on Wheels programs. The local council on aging or local chapter of the Alzheimer's Association should have information about what organization in your area may offer this service.

Find out about the availability of neighborhood teenagers,

adult neighbors, friends, family members, volunteers from religious or social organizations, housekeepers, and companions. For anyone you are considering having come in to help, observe whether she seems able to communicate with the person with Alzheimer's. The helper must seem to enjoy being around the patient, not frustrated or bored.

Introduce the helper in a way that doesn't leave the patient feeling as if he is the problem. "Joyce is here to help me get some things done," you might say. Don't leave the helper immediately with the patient — give him time to adjust to this new situation. If the patient seems to be acting up, stay in the room with the patient and helper several times, making the experience positive for everyone. Recognize that you may have to postpone your own plans at times to make sure that the patient is comfortable with the helper.

Asking family members and friends to help out can present certain complications. First, be honest, letting the person know exactly what is happening with the Alzheimer's patient, and explain that you need help on a regular basis — every Tuesday afternoon between two and five o'clock, for example — not "when you're able to come." The commitment has to be pleasurable for all concerned in some way. If the family member thinks this responsibility is a chore, the patient will know that. In such a case, it is far better to pay the teenager next door, who is willing to be polite and helpful for a few hours, to help out.

If a helper doesn't arrive on schedule, talk openly and honestly about the situation. "How can I meet your needs, since this doesn't seem to be working?" If the problems can't be resolved, you will have to replace the no-show with a helper who is more reliable.

What about seeking volunteer helpers from religious or social organizations? Good helpers of this sort are generally hard to find. Either the volunteers have no experience or they have little interest in dealing with someone with Alzheimer's. And if the patient, while attending a service or event, has been disruptive, the volunteer may feel alienated from him.

You may want to look for other organizations that can help out. Home health care agencies should be able to provide aides, nursing assistants, visiting nurses, companions, and housekeepers to help in matters such as:

- Personal care of the patient (bathing and dressing)
- Laundry services
- Escorting to medical appointments
- Light housekeeping
- Preparing meals
- Companionship (both in the home and in social settings)
- Case management (see page 172)

After determining the type of services the patient will need, try to find someone who is trained in taking care of Alzheimer's patients. Most home health care workers do not have this training, but you may be able to learn about agencies with trained personnel by calling your local chapter of the Alzheimer's Association, speaking with other care partners, or looking through the list of organizations in Further Resources, page 212. Here are the most common kinds of home helpers:

- Visiting nurse. comes to the house at a physician's request. The visiting nurse can perform most medical procedures that a doctor specifies — changing dressings, giving injections, performing physical therapy, and so forth. Note that this may be the only helper who is covered by Medicare/Medicaid; be sure to ask if outside insurance will cover the requested helper's services.
- Certified nursing assistant or aide: can do minor medical tasks such as changing bandages on scratches and scrapes, putting on leg braces, and assisting with bedpans or urinals

(be sure to find out the differences between "certified" and "uncertified" assistants, which will vary by state). Aides "cannot" (that is, they are not supposed to) give medications, although, as a practical matter, most do so.

- Nursing assistant or nurse's aide: can do personal care tasks, such as washing a patient.
- Companion: sits with the patient and provides companionship, takes him for walks, to restaurants, or movies; does not do cooking or cleaning.
- Housekeeper: does light housekeeping (does not clean refrigerators, gutters, or windows, for example); does not provide patient care.

Here's a checklist to think about when interviewing a home health care agency:

- Will the same helper come every time? (It's best for an Alzheimer's patient to see a familiar person. Any agreement should specify that the agency will send the same person each time.)
- Are the agency's personnel bonded? This helps guarantee higher quality of service and reduces the risk of theft and other concerns. Of course, you cannot be completely assured of a helper's honesty. Get references, if possible, and don't leave money, jewelry, or other valuables around.
- How long has the agency been serving the community? Length of time is often a good indication of the organization's reputation. (But keep in mind that new agencies open because of the lack of competent agencies.)
- How does the agency handle emergencies? Are some staff members on duty, or at least available, at all times?
- What services will they charge for?
- What supplies will they charge for?
- Has Medicare approved the agency?

- Will any governmental assistance (such as Medicare or Medicaid) pay for needed items?
- Will the agency be in regular contact with the patient's physician?
- Can the patient and habilitator help decide the patient's plan of care?
- Does the agency teach family members how to carry out the types of care it gives? If the agency person transfers the patient from bath to bed, for example, she needs to teach the family how to do this as well.
- Does the supervisor make regular visits to the home? Who at the agency checks to be sure that the services/supplies are being provided as promised?
- Who is the contact person for questions or concerns?

If the helper you hire through an agency is not trained in working with Alzheimer's patients, explain the five tenets of habilitation to him and emphasize how this approach makes the experience work better for everyone.

You'll know within a few weeks whether the helper you've hired is not working (if the house or the patient is repeatedly not clean, for example). Watch the patient's body language — notice if she is frowning a lot or acting more assertive or aggressive. If the helper is not doing his or her job, the person with Alzheimer's may be trying to communicate her displeasure. Sometimes even the nicest helper isn't the right person if he reminds the patient of someone else. If matters do not appear to be going well, check whether a symptom of the disease is causing the problem; the patient might make false accusations out of paranoia, for example.

If all goes well, the services of a home health care agency can be a godsend, providing the care partner a badly needed respite. The agency personnel can show you useful techniques for dealing with an Alzheimer's patient and can serve as a sounding board as you develop a plan of care. And if one aide doesn't work out, the agency should be able to provide you with another — which can be easier than advertising in the classifieds or trying to find someone through a network of friends and colleagues.

Care Partnering in Your Home, Not the Patient's

If you do not live with the patient, you may think about caring for him in your home. Bringing a person with Alzheimer's into a home with other family members presents a unique set of challenges that you need to consider ahead of time. First, have an open, honest conversation with everyone who lives with you about the situation. Do your family members genuinely like the person? If you have children, explain that the patient may act differently from other people. Several great books and videos about people with Alzheimer's are available (see Further Resources, page 217). Engage children in the discussion so that they can feel vested in the decision.

Another matter to consider before asking a patient to live with you is the need to modify your house, which may be time-consuming and financially draining. Keep in mind that an Alzheimer's patient requires plenty of space for perceptual reasons, as well as a room to himself: a small residence simply will not make sense. And if the house is shared by a number of people, the distractions may be overwhelming to the patient.

If you have a job, it may be difficult, if not impossible, to care properly for the person with Alzheimer's. Will your job allow you to leave unexpectedly if you need to? How often can you do that? And if you can't leave work to take care of an emergency, is someone else available to help? Overall, will your job be conducive to the home routine you'll have to develop?

Having an Alzheimer's patient in your home will definitely affect the neighborhood as well. She may act erratically or have a variety of behavioral problems that neighbors may find troubling or embarrassing. You should be prepared to communicate with your neighbors about the patient; reluctance to discuss the situation may cause discomfiture. You could write a letter alerting your neighbors to the likelihood of some irrational behavior. You might say, "My mother has come to live with us. She has Alzheimer's. If she walks into your house without knocking or does something that makes you uncomfortable, please welcome her in and call us immediately. Here's our phone number."

As soon as you have decided to bring the patient into your home, seek financial and elder-care legal counseling. If the person owns the residence where he has lived up until now, it may have to be sold to help pay for his care. According to the Alzheimer's Association, as of 2001, the cost of caring for a person with Alzheimer's was approximately $12,500 per year. Also make sure that the proper clauses concerning physical and medical matters are inserted into documents such as the power of attorney.

The decision to bring a patient into your home doesn't have to be a permanent one. If at some point the family no longer wants to keep the person at home, other arrangements can be made.

Share-Care

Share-care is one of the most helpful options available to primary care partners. Generally, two or three care partners in a support group will organize a schedule for having one person look after several Alzheimer's patients for a given period of time, in exchange for another person looking after them at another set time. This not only gives care partners time to relax, but it's a wonderful bonding experience with other care partners, since these people really understand your situation. And they can speak frankly if the situation is not working well. "Your wife's nice," I once heard someone say to another care partner, "but she's peeing in my petunias. I think we'll have to make other arrangements."

In most cases, share-care arrangements simply happen — someone mentions it in the support group, and the care partners work out the plan. Often support-group participants are from the same geographic area and have similar work and ethnic backgrounds, which makes it easier for the care partners to understand each other, and allows the patients to feel more comfortable in someone else's home. Share-care shouldn't begin on the first day of the support group, however — the care partners must learn to know and like each other and learn one another's fears and concerns.

To set up a share-care arrangement, first arrange a meeting for care partners and patients. Everyone must like and trust each other.

Case Management Program

When a patient cannot live with a local care partner, family members generally hire a case manager — a social worker — to organize and manage the afflicted person's plan of care. The local council on aging, which is state-run and thus has guidelines, is the best place to find a high-quality case management program. The Case Management Society of America produces a directory and Web site that lists case managers by state (see Further Resources, page 214).

Initially the case manager goes into the home of the person with Alzheimer's and does a complete assessment of the patient and the home, focusing on safety issues, environmental concerns, financial matters, and the like. The case manager can arrange for the services of a home health care agency, as well as for financial and legal services, personal emergency response systems, home-delivered meals from Meals on Wheels, and much more.

A case management program is ideal for a patient who wants to remain living at home for as long as possible, and perhaps through the entire course of the disease. Depending on the patient's income, Medicare and Medicaid may pay for the services. Long-term insurance may also cover them, if they keep the patient from having to enter a nursing home.

A downside to case management can be the cost, which may

range from several hundred dollars a week for individual services to fifty thousand dollars a year for full-time care. In addition, the patient may experience a sense of having lost control. A good case manager tries to keep the patient feeling that she is still part of the decision-making, however.

Generally, early-stage patients welcome case management programs. If the person with dementia can cognitively grasp that the program will allow her to stay at home, she is likely to cooperate well with the case manager.

Adult Day Health and Day Care Centers

Another workable alternative for patients in the later early stage and middle stage of Alzheimer's is an adult day health or day care program. Adult day health centers provide enrichment activities outside the home. These centers have trained staff and a trained nurse on the premises. Adult day care centers are similar, but are not required to have a trained staff or nurse available.

Be sure that the adult day health program staff is thoroughly trained in interacting with people with dementia. A well-run program can offer the habilitator a respite by providing meals as well as hours of structured programming — including bathing and naps, if necessary. Since filling leisure time is often a difficulty for the patient, a program that provides fun, socialization, and chances for success makes sense. It may not be the best choice for patients who are not functioning well, however, and could lead to greater depression if the afflicted person spends a lot of time with patients who exhibit signs of more advanced dementia. It is also not appropriate for very late-stage Alzheimer's patients — these programs should not be considered a "sitting" service.

Bruce's family had a meeting and decided that three days a week in an adult day health program would enrich his life with activities that were both physically and mentally rewarding. After entering the program, the seventy-eight-year-old became much more engaged and interested in everything. On his "home" days, he wanted to go on walks with his hired companion. He never seemed to remember exactly what he did at the day program, but when asked, he would respond, "Whatever it was, it was great."

Bruce's family was fortunate that he remained outgoing and open to new possibilities. Many care partners, however, find that convincing an Alzheimer's patient to go to an adult day health program is difficult at first, since change seems threatening and confusing. Here are some techniques that can make the move more comfortable for both patient and habilitator.

When introducing the topic, explain to the patient that the adult day health program needs him rather than saying he needs the program. If he is still functioning well, you may be able to convince him that the center needs a volunteer helper who will help the staff by setting up meals and programs, transporting people in wheelchairs, reading poetry, or directing sing-alongs. If this explanation fails, or when it is no longer sufficient, explain that you need time to accomplish chores around the house, go shopping, work, or garden, and his attendance in a program will make that possible.

Set a time limit on how long the person with Alzheimer's will attend the center; you might say, "Let's do it just for this week because I have something to do." The following week, you can repeat the same request. Be persistent and confident that the program is a positive choice for the patient — even if she doesn't believe it. Staff members are accustomed to dealing with resistant patients and are quite adept at changing the negative into the positive.

If the patient hesitates when he arrives at the center, be sure to have a trained staff member actually move him into the facility each day. Have the staff person meet you at the car if you're driving to the facility, or have the bus driver meet you at your door. Staff people are trained to deal with reluctant patients, and a patient will often more willingly go with one of them than with the care partner or another family member. If the patient refuses to get dressed, send him in pajamas. The centers are equipped for such situations.

Have the center take photographs or videos of the patient having a good time at the program. When she insists, at day's end, that she had a terrible time and won't go back, the photograph will remind her how much fun the program was and will ease your mind about sending her there.

13

Receiving Care Outside
of a Family Home

*Good decisions are born
out of fears overcome
and baggage left behind.*

MAL, EIGHTY-TWO years old and in the middle stage of Alzheimer's, lived with her daughter's family, which included two teenage grandchildren. Long before Mal was diagnosed, her daughter and son-in-law decided that they should always take care of her. Recently, when one of the grandchildren had some friends over, Mal walked into the family room clad only in a slip and boisterously exclaimed, "Prisoners, prisoners, peaches!" Clearly agitated, she shook the front doorknob, trying to get out of the house.

Later that night, Mal's daughter heard the two kids huddled together on the porch, talking about the "totally awful embarrassment" their grandmother had caused. "What are we going to do?" one said. "I don't want her to be here anymore — she's ruining everything." The other seemed equally upset. "I stay away from this wacko house as much as possible. Mom and Dad just keep saying they promised they'd always take care of Nana. But what about us?"

Mal's social ineptness, lack of inhibition and judgment, and difficulty with language are typical manifestations of middle-stage Alzheimer's. The negative body language of her grandchildren most likely confused her even more. At that point, for the sake of the family, Mal should have been moved to a setting designed to care for people with Alzheimer's disease. The family could visit for brief periods, contributing to Mal's care but focusing primarily on positive family interactions. In this more appropriate setting, everyone in the family would have been happier, better off, and, ideally, free of guilt and denial.

Consider the story of Michael and Jennifer, too. After their mother died, they sincerely promised their father, Renato, that they would take care of him in his own home "forever." Renato had cared for his wife at home and now he expected his children to do the same for him. No one expected, or planned for, Alzheimer's. But as the disease progressed, Renato's inability to live alone forced caregiving issues. Who would cook for him? Who would make sure he took his medication? Michael had troubles of his own that made it impossible for him to care for his father, and he began phoning Jennifer daily, begging her to take Renato into her home. "But he won't leave his home — and I promised him he could stay," Jennifer would cry, feeling powerless to go against her father's wishes even in the face of dementia. She tried to reassure herself, saying "He'll be okay. I stop by every day. I keep the doors locked. I bring him pizza. What more can I do? He doesn't want to leave. He sits and watches TV all day. But it's his life."

Then one night Renato, locked in his home alone, awoke in the chair in front of the TV, where he now slept every night, and shuffled into the kitchen. He turned on the burner under the teakettle sitting on the stove, returned to his chair, and fell back to sleep. The teakettle burned dry, then the papers on the kitchen counter caught fire and spread to curtains, cabinets, walls. Renato woke up to the wail of the smoke alarms, although he did not understand what the sound was. Seeing the fire, he cowered near the locked front door, where the fire department found him, suffering from smoke inhalation. Had they arrived a few minutes later, Renato would not have survived.

As the progression of their father's disease caused changes in his need for care, Michael and Jennifer's plans for him also had to change, even if they felt guilt-ridden for making that decision. If having Renato live with one of his children was out of the question, engaging the services of a visiting nurse, sending him to an adult day center, or placing him in a nursing home would have been appropriate options. And the decision would have been made out of love for the parent — not out of guilt.

Families rally more easily when a parent requires a short-term hospital stay for an acute problem. Long-term — or, perhaps more aptly, "lifespan" — care, however, presents more difficult choices. Plans need to be continually revisited and revised. Promises — to both the patient and other family members — can be fulfilled only if circumstances warrant it, and promises should not be made and kept out of guilt.

Many children have assured parents that they would never be sent to a nursing home. Such a promise — made at a time when the parents were cognitively intact and able to care for themselves — leaves the children riddled with guilt when, after trying everything else, placement in a nursing home seems the only option. It's extraordinarily distressing to feel you've failed to care for your parent or to feel you've broken your promise to the parent or other family members. Consequently — and perhaps too often unavoidably — the parent remains in a less appropriate setting or receives less than optimal care for far too long, all because of a promise made before the disease had progressed or had been properly diagnosed.

Promises made to others when the situation was simpler may be impossible to keep after Alzheimer's intrudes and causes tremendous changes. Disease complicates the decisions and necessitates new plans. Use love as your guide: *Do I love her enough, am I worried enough about her well-being, to have her be angry with me for a while if someone else can care for her better than I can?* For many patients and their families, home care is not the ideal option — everyone may be better able to thrive if the patient lives outside the family home.

If you are caring for a patient in your home, you'll know that the time has come to relinquish care when you go out to do an errand and no longer want to go back into the house when you return — that is, when the negative feelings of being with the patient fully outweigh the positives. Practicing the tenets of habilitation is impossible without love, trust, and comfort. You cannot successfully reassure and comfort the patient if you don't have the sensitivity born of these feelings. When that time comes, you need to have already chosen the next steps to take.

The following options can, if properly selected, allow a person with Alzheimer's to live with dignity and self-respect:

- Group home/foster-care setting: Several people with Alzheimer's living together in a primary caregiver's home.
- Assisted-living center: An establishment for patients (and their spouses) who require minimal assistance but need some help with directions and activities of daily living.
- Alzheimer's assisted-living center: An establishment designed to meet the needs of Alzheimer's patients (and their spouses).
- Nursing home: An establishment for patients with advanced psychosocial and medical needs.
- Special-care unit: A designated area in an assisted-living center or nursing home, set apart for people with progressive dementia.

Each of these support systems offers differing possibilities to allow both patient and habilitator to thrive rather than merely mark time.

Group Home/Foster-Care Setting

In a group home, several people with Alzheimer's live together in a primary caregiver's home. This wonderful, but fairly rare, situation typically comes about when family members who have kept a loved one at home have extra space and invite others to live with them for a fee.

Group homes usually have five or six people living together; each patient has his own room, and they share a living room, dining room, and kitchen. The setting is like a regular home except that a family member (or sometimes a professional staff person) sleeps in the house overnight. The care partners are usually trained to work with Alzheimer's patients and help create Alzheimer's-friendly activities, chores, and outings. This is as close to home care as possible.

The habilitation techniques discussed in this book are perfectly suited to this care option: patients have a great opportunity to feel successful, and the entire house can be modified for maximum comfort. In one house I helped design, we painted each patient's bedroom a different vibrant color — making the room easily recognizable, comfortable, and personalized. Each resident can spend time alone in her own room, yet other people are nearby for socializing, which helps alleviate feelings of loneliness and isolation. The care for each resident can be personalized; each can have his own schedule and routine.

Unfortunately, group homes are not funded through any third-party source — they are paid for only on a private-pay basis, and the costs can be prohibitive. If a group home is available to you, find out the costs up front, and be sure that they can be checked and detailed in the future. Make sure the care provider isn't just trying to make money by taking in patients — he or she should be properly trained and should understand the particular needs of people with Alzheimer's. Talk to family members of other residents; ask for references, and check with the local Better Business Bureau.

Assisted-Living Center

Assisted-living centers are for elders (and their spouses) who require minimal assistance with directions, bathing, meal preparation, medications, and so forth. Alzheimer's assisted-living centers are designed to meet the needs of Alzheimer's patients who are not ready for nursing home placement.

To assess an assisted-living facility, consider the following factors:

- Convenient location: Will family and friends be able to visit on a regular schedule?
- Facility tour: Can you drop by for a tour anytime, or does the management insist on a guided tour? You should be able to see the facility from the resident's perspective at any time. A staff guide will point out areas or programs that you may miss if touring unescorted.
- Patient control: Will the Alzheimer's patient be safe from the dangers of wandering into other areas of the building or on the grounds? Have security and emergency systems, such as door alarms or security cameras, been installed?
- Training: Is the staff trained specifically to interact with Alzheimer's residents? Local chapters or the National Alzheimer's Association can provide brochures for education of staff — see Special-Care Unit, below, for more details.
- Staff: Do staff members appear to enjoy their work interacting with residents? Does the staffing ratio assure individual attention and care? There should be at least one staff person for eight to twelve residents. Is the staff friendly toward you?
- Odor: A pervasive unpleasant odor can be an indicator of unsanitary conditions. (However, an offensive odor outside a patient's room is generally indicative of an accident and may not indicate poor housekeeping.)

- Common areas: Are they well designed and inviting, allowing for socialization? Are chairs comfortable and facing each other, making the space conducive to conversation?
- Private areas: Are the patients encouraged to personalize their rooms with memorabilia and photographs?
- All areas: Is the environment specifically designed for Alzheimer's patients rather than outsiders?
- Activity programs: Are the activity programs of interest to the Alzheimer's patient?
- Outside activities: Are there opportunities and areas for outdoor activities?
- Family involvement: Does the center ask for the family's involvement in formulating its plan of care?
- Food: Is the food appetizing, nutritious, and suitable for the declining skills of Alzheimer's residents? (See Chapter 8.)
- References: Will the facility provide names and contact information for family members of other residents?
- Peer interaction: If the Alzheimer's patients are intermingled with other residents, do these people sometimes treat dementia patients with less friendliness and support than they treat other people? Talk about this with other families of Alzheimer's patients.

It is important to consult with a financial planner before moving a person to an assisted-living center. You may too quickly spend down funds that will be needed later, when the patient needs to move to a more professional setting, for example. Also, assisted living may be suitable for Alzheimer's patients for only a short term. And moving again as the disease progresses can be traumatizing for both patient and care partner.

But assisted-living facilities provide a safety net for thousands of Alzheimer's patients who would otherwise fall into a gaping hole of residential care. These centers promote continued independence and provide enrichment possibilities for early-stage patients. Because residents bring their own furniture, the transition from home is often easier, and as the disease progresses, familiar surroundings can be a great comfort. Also, the companionship of other residents can be a godsend for care partner and patient.

Nursing Home

When Kristen was making plans to place her father-in-law, Mel, in a nursing home, she told her support group of her feelings of failure. "I feel that I'm abandoning him in some way. They don't know him the way I do or my husband does."

Kristen needed to keep in mind the reasons that prompted her to seek an alternative living arrangement. Mel had begun to need more care than Kristen, the mother of three young children, could handle. Although her husband tried to be helpful, he was disturbed to see his dad in decline, and there was less and less interaction between the two. Mel was wandering away from home several times a week and had aggressively threatened Kristen when she tried to stop him. Moreover, none of her husband's siblings had offered assistance. In short, there had been no other choice than to find good professional care.

The support group gave Kristen the reassurance she needed. They viewed her decision to place Mel in a good nursing home as an act of love, giving him a safe setting where wandering wasn't an issue and where his frustration and anxiety could be reduced. Also, the staff worked eight-hour shifts, which meant that every worker could return refreshed. Kristen's future visits with Mel would be warm and meaningful, and she could enjoy a more fulfilling life with her family.

At some point in the care-partnering process, the best way to care for the patient may be to relinquish some of the responsibility to the professional staff of a nursing home. Too often, family members seek a nursing home bed at a moment of crisis rather

184 • BEYOND HABILITATION

than planning this move thoroughly ahead of time. Planning such a move with the patient can also be beneficial by conveying trust in his remaining control and willingness to have him participate in the process.

The variety of names describing these facilities can be confusing. The most common terms, depending on the geographical area you live in, are nursing care or health care centers, nursing homes, rest homes, foster-care homes, adult-care centers or homes, Alzheimer's centers, or special-care units. The latter two categories are set up to care only for folks diagnosed with Alzheimer's or other progressive dementias. I discuss them in the following section.

Nursing homes have come a long way in offering care to people with various kinds of dementia. Many, however, have not come far enough; it is necessary to visit, tour, and ask questions of people both inside and outside of the facility. If you have any doubts about a facility, check with the council on aging, your local department of public health, police department, Better Business Bureau, and people in the neighborhood. After all, you are choosing a home for someone you care about; if you plan ahead, you should be able to have more than a single choice.

Placing the person with Alzheimer's in a good nursing home can leave you with feelings of ease and satisfaction, knowing that she is being given care perhaps better than you could provide. You can still have positive visits and provide ongoing love. Although long-term-care facilities vary greatly from community to community, some basic features should be present in the one you choose. Ideally, try to find a special-care unit (see page 189). But even these units vary greatly, ranging from locked wards all the way to completely habilitative programs. Be sure to obtain and read, early on, the Alzheimer's Association pamphlet on choosing a long-term-care setting (see the Alzheimer's Association listing in Further Resources, page 212).

When assessing a nursing home, consider the points listed above for assisted-living centers as well as the following:

- Family council meetings: Ask if the facility offers meetings run by the families of residents who are not able to speak for themselves, and without staff members present. These meetings allow families to collectively voice concerns and ideas. A trusted staff member may act as liaison between the group and administration. For those residents who are able to speak for themselves, a residents' council should be in place. Ask if the facility holds such meetings regularly, and perhaps ask to attend one.

- Family support: Unlike family councils, which discuss concerns about the facility, family support groups discuss the emotional side of dealing with Alzheimer's, and the meetings are led by a facilitator. Studies have shown that family support groups are often extraordinarily beneficial to families and patients alike. If such a group meets regularly, attend a meeting or two to see if you want to participate.

- Medical director: Do you approve of the medical director? This person makes the final decisions about your loved one's medical care. Does she have a reputation in the community as an advocate for people with Alzheimer's? Ask other residents' families what interaction they have had with her.

- State survey: Ask to see the latest state survey report on the facility; this is public information and should be readily available. The department that handles this responsibility (whose name is usually a variation of public health department) makes yearly assessments of any facility that accepts Medicare or Medicaid patients. The report is available for public viewing. The facility should get the highest grade; if not, the administrator should be able to easily explain the few deficiencies, and there should be demonstrable proof that efforts are being made to correct the issues.

- Medicaid: Does the nursing home accept Medicaid payments? Many don't. When all of the patient's funds have been expended, Medicaid will pay for nursing home care.

Don't settle for the first nursing home you find nearby — tour several and take notes. Drop in unexpectedly. Listen to your gut instincts. Often when a family tours a facility, they come away with a certain feeling about the place. The feeling may be negative, but not necessarily. A good facility will feel warm and homelike because the interaction between staff and residents is friendly, and the philosophy of the nursing home is obviously positive in all aspects, from dietary programs to administration.

As soon as Alzheimer's has been diagnosed, you should formulate legal plans for eventual long-term care. Consult an attorney or accountant who specializes in these issues, and see Chapter 3 for further information on powers of attorney and living wills. Few insurance policies cover nursing home placement. Many people with Alzheimer's or other progressive dementias have been duped into believing that "long-term-care insurance" will cover their situation. It usually does not. *Read the fine print carefully to be sure that "cognitive" disease or "mental incapacity" or "dementia" is not excluded.* Some states have special programs to help cover *some* costs of *some* care in assisted-living facilities, foster homes, retirement centers, and nursing homes. Check with your state's department of elder services. Medicare will help pay for some services.

The actual moment of bringing the person to the nursing home can be painful, but it need not be terrible. First, before the patient arrives, take some of her personal effects to her new room, so that familiar items will be waiting. Make sure clothing is in the drawers, favorite mementos are on the shelves, and so forth. The patient shouldn't arrive with a suitcase, as if he were going on a trip. Most important is that the new room possess a familiar odor associated with home — his brand of shaving cream, for example, or soap.

Have the aide or another person who will be spending much of the day with the patient (ask ahead of time who it will be) greet him at the door. Let that person take over the social dynamics, showing the patient around and introducing the other residents. Staff members do this regularly and know how to do it properly.

If the patient doesn't want to get out of the car, let the staff take over. Often the person with Alzheimer's is exercising control over the care partner — expressing anger or frustration may be her way of communicating her displeasure to you. Although she doesn't know the staff members, she doesn't have a past history with them, either, so she may not need to assert that she is still "in charge." The act of entering a nursing home, of being taken over by competent, professional staff, may actually be a tremendous relief, but the patient may not want to admit it.

When you get to the patient's room, stay for half an hour or so, then come up with a reason for having to leave. Figure out a reason ahead of time. If it's around lunchtime, have lunch with him, kiss him goodbye in the lunchroom, and leave. Discuss your leaving plan ahead of time with the staff. If the patient is angry, that is not necessarily a bad sign — it's a normal reaction. Her negativity will dissipate as time goes on and as she grows accustomed to the facility.

When the patient who has been sharing a home with a care partner moves into a nursing home, the care partner is very likely to feel guilty about relinquishing an essential part of loving (nurturing), or she may worry that others will see it that way. Even if the need for placement is clear, the action can be a powerful blow to the habilitator's self-esteem. Also, nursing home placement can lead to feelings of competition with the staff. If you have any of these reactions, look upon this change as an opportunity to share care.

After you place the patient in a professional home, the best way to care for yourself may be to take some time to rejuvenate and realize how important your role has been and continues to be in the overall care package. Most facilities will suggest that you take some time away from the patient to adjust, and allow the new resident to do the same. Four or five days should be enough time for the patient to become somewhat adapted to new surroundings and faces, while you catch up on needed relaxation. Telephone calls may help keep contact with the patient, who may have been told that you are temporarily out of town — a fiblet to help the adjustment.

Now that someone else is sharing the care, make the most of your visits to the patient's new home (remember that the nursing home *is* his home now). Check the schedule of activities or enrichment programs and arrange to visit when the person will not be involved in these periods of socialization. Plan to visit for half an hour to an hour, a long enough time for positive interaction without interfering with the patient's new routine. Keep in mind that he may simply stop paying attention to you.

Offering information about your loved one will help nursing staff and other professional caregivers connect with the patient through her long-term memories. Her previous routine should become the basis for the new plan of care. Making sure that the staff knows the patient's likes, dislikes, and food preferences will make the adjustment more pleasant. Hobbies can be started right away as part of a personalized recreational program. Physical activity is still important; when you visit, take her for a walk outside or around the facility. She needs familiar faces as much as ever, so encourage family and friends to visit, but to do so one at a time to lower the level of stimulation.

You can take to the nursing home a number of items that the patient will enjoy. For instance, he may like listening to an audiotape of family members' voices (label the tape and be sure the staff keeps track of it). You can take some favorite foods. (Again, label these, then put them in a refrigerator at the nursing home.) Take photo albums that the two of you can browse through during your visit. (If you plan to leave the albums with staff members, label the pictures. Then the staff can mention the descriptions as they peruse them with the patient.)

If you want to take the patient out of the home for a few hours, a whole day, or a weekend, follow the advice of the staff on whether that is a good idea. Then check in with them a few hours after you return to gauge the advisability of future ventures. Going out may prove more complicated than you think, as Hunter found out.

Hunter insisted on taking his brother Jerry, who had been in his assisted-living facility for only two weeks, out for a Sunday drive and an ice cream cone. When they returned, the two brothers shared a bear hug, and Hunter was sure that everything had gone well.

But on the way back to his room, Jerry saw the large grandfather clock. "It's six o'clock. Where's my supper?" he demanded.

"I'll see what I can find for you," the young assistant said.

"Find for me! I want a supper like everyone else. And now, now, now!"

Jerry's overreaction, a first for him, occurred because the outing had confused and disoriented him. He was trying hard to exercise control over something in his life, and it might as well be a meal. The staff suggested that Hunter visit with his brother at the facility for the time being.

Learning to communicate and work with the staff will help make the experience better for everyone.

Special-Care Unit (SCU)

A special-care unit is an area within an assisted-living facility, nursing home, or other health care facility specifically intended for people with progressive dementia. These units vary from facility to facility. An SCU may be no different from the rest of the facility except for being behind locked doors. Or it may have a special philosophy, well-trained and plentiful staff, and an environment that meets the specific needs of patients with Alzheimer's. (The Alzheimer's Association chapter in your area may be able to point out the better SCUs.)

When assessing a special-care unit, use the guidelines listed above for nursing homes, but expect to find considerably more information relating to programming, training, philosophy, and design. When I look at a special-care unit for program integrity, I am hoping to find:

- A mission statement specific to the unit and understood by every staff member. For example: *Our mission is to live in the residents' world and to try to hear what they are* not *saying.*
- Only patients with an admission diagnosis of Alzheimer's disease or a related dementia.
- Use of preadmission assessment and social history as the backbone for developing a specialized plan of care for each resident.
- Availability of physical, occupational, and speech therapies.
- All staff trained to work with patients with Alzheimer's in a program either offered or approved by the local chapter of the National Alzheimer's Association.
- Consistent staff assigned to the SCU only, with coverage twenty-four hours a day, seven days a week, assuring the same resident-to-staff ratio every day.
- Assigned activity staff (as opposed to regular staff) working only on the SCU every day, seven days a week.
- An outdoor area designated specifically for SCU residents and not used by other residents of the facility, so the Alzheimer's patients don't mix with people who do not understand their behavior.
- A quality assurance committee to ensure that problems are recognized, evaluated, and dealt with.
- A community volunteer program of people who regularly visit patients one to one or put on special programs such as musical performances or pet visits.
- A program director who oversees the philosophy, training, and support of staff, residents, and families.
- A behavior team that meets regularly to ensure that habilita-

tion approaches are used and that residents are not routinely medicated for behavior control.

- Infrequent use of behavior medications, such as antidepressants, antianxiety drugs, mood elevators and stabilizers, and antipsychotics. In a good SCU, only 10 percent of patients will be taking such medications at any time. All pharmaceuticals should be used for short periods only and should be reevaluated frequently.)

- Counseling services for residents and families, and possibly for the community, to help develop coping skills.

- Ongoing assessments to monitor changes related to Alzheimer's disease and create individualized programs and daily care.

- Team meetings held whenever necessary to discuss patient changes.

- Family involvement in recreational programs and family council meetings that provide input to the staff on behalf of the residents, who can no longer articulate their concerns.

- Attention to environmental design, including the use of color to identify and define spatial area and aid in way-finding; flooring that helps walking and reduces confusion; easily interpreted wall hangings that can be touched and handled; and acoustics that help residents process information by decreasing noise stimulation.

- A finger food menu.

- Secured doors monitored by a nonintrusive system (no loud alarms).

- Most important, happy residents interacting positively with happy staff.

You may not find all these items in your evaluation, but they provide a baseline for comparing different SCUs. A pervasive feeling of comfort and well-being can mean as much as or more than other, more tangible factors.

I am not a Pollyanna. I consider myself a card-carrying realist, leavened with a bit of altruism. I do not believe that every care-partnering relationship will turn into an idyllic situation. Some families are much better in a crisis, rallying to support their loved one during an acute hospital stay, than they are when faced with the complex problems of long-term care.

But all families will do far better when the considerations of lifespan care are dealt with on the basis of realistic assessments rather than on guilt. Most important, if families follow the tenets of habilitation, the result will be a far more positive collaboration that will enrich the lives of all concerned.

14

Inspiration

I played as a child.
I danced when I was young.
I laughed yesteryear.
Today, I recall
the games, the music, the joy
over and over and over again.

IN 2001 I ATTENDED the annual Public Policy Forum sponsored by the National Alzheimer's Association, and as always it was a wonderful experience. Every year a great many people with Alzheimer's from all fifty states attend the meeting, as do thousands of other people, including care partners, professionals, and legislators. The patients who spoke at the 2001 conference were nervous and often fearful. They were poignant in their silence as they collected words for their next sentence. But they were also passionate about their concerns, willing to share their personal stories, and eager to participate in life.

The audience gave a standing ovation to these heroes. Even more accolades should go to the many thousands of patients who speak at other conferences, talk about their lives on television shows, walk in Alzheimer's marathons, or write newspaper articles and letters to legislators. Acclaim should also go to patients who make videos to influence public policy, appear on educational panels, give college lectures on the disease, speak to school-age children, and, in the early stages of the disease, volunteer to help Meals on Wheels programs, or work in hospitals or nursing home activity programs, reading poetry, working on craft programs, playing the piano, and so forth.

People living with Alzheimer's are amazing, and talking to them can be helpful for anyone who faces becoming a care partner of someone with the disease. Patients continually remind us that they need us to recognize their determination, bolster their sense of self-worth, and provide appropriate support throughout the course of the disease. As I've emphasized throughout this book, care partners should recognize patients' remaining skills and create a positive emotional environment in which these skills may be used. Such a setting enables patients to feel successful, have good interactions, and maintain a sense of dignity. Patients say they want these three outcomes as they live daily with Alzheimer's.

Consider the comments of three remarkable people I know who have repeatedly inspired me as they live with this disease.

My friend Bernard Reisman, a former chair of the department of Jewish studies at Brandeis University, told me of both the sadness that living with Alzheimer's has brought him and his resolve to maintain his sense of self-worth. An eloquent man, whose bright eyes and wonderful smile transcend his professorial tones, Bernie always considered himself a role model and authority for his children and grandchildren and a mentor to students. His realization that he was losing hold of these positions made him sad.

"I don't know what I'll do when my sons no longer come to me for answers," he told me. "I wonder now if they look at me differently. Do they ask someone else for information that they once would have asked me? Will my grandsons ever think of me as a great scholar or just as an old man who repeats himself? I am like the great pitcher who injures his arm. Except that my super body part has been my brain, and now it's injured. Two more strikes and I'm out.

"But I'm not out yet — I'm still at bat. I've always been a fighter, and I sure as hell am not giving up now. You bet I'm sad. And angry, and damn ornery too, but I've learned to listen, and learn, and live for today. I'm trying, I'm trying hard.

"I walk, I play tennis, I swim. I take medications to help Alzheimer's — not to cure it but to ease it a bit. My family and I still travel around the globe. I just finished writing a book with my son. I go to an early-stage support group, and I'm part of the Alzheimer's Association speaker's bureau. I have to continue to teach — it's not easy for me to lecture and it's certainly not the way I used to. I can talk about how to live better with this disease, and no one can shut me up."

In 2002 Bernard Reisman received an honorary degree from American Hebrew University. He also spoke with fervor at a legislative breakfast, pleaded for more research funding at a national Alzheimer's Association annual meeting, appeared on the front page of the *Boston Globe* in a feature article about Alzheimer's, and traveled to Iceland with his wife. Bernie still has much to say and to give.

In 1995 tall, handsome Jim Anthony walked into our early-stage support group. Jim, in his fifties, had just been diagnosed with Alzheimer's and had lost his job because of problems caused by the disease. He had been misdiagnosed several times before that and now felt relieved to know conclusively, through a brain biopsy, that Alzheimer's was the cause of his cognitive problems. Numbers were particularly difficult for Jim; dialing the telephone, balancing his checkbook, and trying to manage appointments left him reeling. His vast lexicon remained intact, however, and he spoke about his daily life fluently and with great humor.

Jim was hungry to learn about habilitative ways that could help him manage his life. Having observed his mother going through Alzheimer's, he was distressed by what was happening to him and by knowing what was to come. But Jim always presented himself to us — and, as I write, still does — as a vital person who is supportive of others. When he spoke to visiting Japanese students at Harvard Medical School in 1997, he made a powerful impression on the audience.

Alzheimer's, he told the group, "used to be a disease that was not discussed. It was considered hopeless. But from a universal perspective, all life is hopeless — in that we all die.

"What is significant about Alzheimer's is that it has the potential to rob us of our understanding. The severity of the disease can be quite daunting. But people with Alzheimer's also work, raise children, go to movies, take vacations, give talks, and refuse to let the disease dictate their lives. People with Alzheimer's disease experience varying degrees of disability. This is not a one-size-fits-all disease.

"One notable dynamic I have observed is that people can become angry with people with Alzheimer's, especially partners and family members. I have seen it in friends, in my family, and in my own experience. The reason for this anger, I suspect, is that Alzheimer's is a frightening disease. One prefers to think that his or her companion is simply not trying hard enough, is being careless, obstinate, difficult, even deliberately trying to provoke his or her partner. And the partner is as puzzled as everyone.

"The anger is something that family members and friends have to own and work through for the sake of the couple, the family, for everyone concerned, even though it is appropriate. A loss of this magnitude cannot be dealt with lightly.

"This does not mean that you cannot laugh. I attend an Alzheimer's support group twice a month, and laughter is an important therapeutic component. Crying is too. We tend to deal with our grief privately. But in a support group, we understand the grief we all share. Our group is remarkable for its spirit of empathy, compassion, and truth-telling. Sometimes we sense that one member of our group is practicing denial. We do not rush in to help him or her get over it, though one or more of us may prod gently. A degree of denial is essential in Alzheimer's. Like someone drinking hot coffee, we sip the truth of our condition carefully and gently.

"One could, of course, rail at the universe, at God, at the physician who diagnosed [him or her]. It is a temptation, and all of us with Alzheimer's have done a bit of that. And adjusting to Alzheimer's is not a stately process like that of a king ascending his throne. It's a bit grubbier than that.

"My mother was diagnosed with Alzheimer's . . . She . . . developed an acceptance of life and its challenges and a wisdom that transcended her limitation. People with Alzheimer's have gifts to give. Do not underestimate their strengths and wisdom. They do not survive Alzheimer's without learning a thing or two.

"I do believe that the afflictions that come to us are nature's way of keeping the planet going. And I do believe that our efforts to sustain life with compassion and common sense are a reflection of our humanity. But we know that our lease on the planet is uncertain. We do celebrate longevity, but we celebrate to a far greater degree those who live well. I am far more interested in living well than in living long, though I am quite willing to hang around for a while. Since I have little control over it, I think I will take it one day at a time."

Jim and his care partner, Bruce, who now live in the Berkshire Hills of western Massachusetts, attend as many Alzheimer's forums and conferences as possible and keep abreast, via computer, of new findings about the disease.

Another outstanding person with Alzheimer's is Shirley Geller, who in 2002 stood before an audience of more than five hundred professionals at a conference in New England on Alzheimer's and spoke about what the disease was like for her. First she described the fears and problems she has encountered, such as recognizing that she will become worse and will have to move to a nursing home someday, that she will repeat questions, lose her ideas in midthought, and have other difficulties. But she also described another side of having Alzheimer's. Her friends have been "extremely supportive and caring," she said, and she felt blessed to have her "wonderful" family, a doctor who had listened to all of her questions, and a "very helpful" support group. "It's important to be able to share problems and concerns with others in the same situation and to have leaders who are able to help with good suggestions," she commented.

"Truthfully, I still enjoy life and get pleasure from it. People are amazed that with this problem, I still have a positive attitude." She concluded, "I am determined to get the most out of each and every day."

Although Bernie, Jim, and Shirley are quite different from one another in personality, social and work history, and disease process, they share many reactions to having Alzheimer's. They feel empowered, their emotions are validated, they live in the here and now, and they feel connected to others.

Having worked with thousands of patients and their families, and having spent many years remembering the meaning, and the emotion, behind the failing words, I want to speak on behalf of the remarkable people who live with progressive dementia. They can show us how to help them, if we listen:

- "Reminding and scolding me does not make me better, only sadder. When someone asks me questions about where I've been and who I've seen and what I did, and I can't retrieve that information, I feel stupid and unworthy."

- "Trying to fill my brain with new ideas and new equipment and new data will not work. My brain is full. Not one speck of space is left for new information to find a seat. If the information can't go in, it can never come out again."

- "Don't wish me out of reverie or worry about my silent times. I still have imaginative explorations to make, and dreams to dream. I have kisses to relive. I have a garden of memories before me, and everything is blooming simultaneously. Don't assume I am sad when I sit alone; most of the time it is the sadness on your face that brings sorrow to my heart."

- "You can make me a part of this world only if you actively involve me, if your connection with me remains until the end. You must constantly reach out and touch me — physically, spiritually, emotionally."
- "You are the conduit to my failing world, a world that has so many possibilities to be filled with laughter, a few shared tears, and memories."

Having spent three decades in the world of the memory-impaired, I am emphatic about the profound change a habilitative care partner can make in the life of an affected person. I am equally sure that the habilitative approach provides the best care for the care partner, because this philosophy helps eliminate confrontation and unnecessary stress. In the end, care partners realize how much stronger they feel as they watch their loved ones relax, with dignity intact.

Habilitation gives us the gift of the present moment. We can speak the language of Alzheimer's, a nonverbal language that transcends illness. With the habilitative approach we can know, in our spirit and our heart, that we have done the best we could — that we have offered the patient chances to be successful, and that both of us can feel worthy.

Glossary

Appendix:
Good Food for People with Alzheimer's

Further Resources

Index

■   ■   ■

Glossary

Alzheimer's disease behavior log: A record of data on a patient's problematic behavior, including time of day, location, and environmental factors, in order to determine the cause of the behavior. (See page 119.)

Activities of daily living (ADL): The basic daily activities, including bathing, dressing, eating, toileting, and sleeping, that health professionals use to judge an Alzheimer's person's need for assistance with physical care.

Busy apron: A plain carpenter's or chef's apron to which various small objects and notions have been attached to occupy the patient. (See page 93.)

Care partner: The person who works with the Alzheimer's patient, providing habilitative cueing, supervision, assistance, and emotional, physical, and cognitive support through the changing stages of the disease.

Contrasting visual field: A light background against which dark objects can be clearly seen or a dark background against which light-colored objects will be more distinct.

Excess disability: A patient's inability to perform certain activities of daily living as a result of having had too much assistance when he was still able to perform those activities. (See page 37.)

Fine motor skills: Physical abilities requiring the use of small muscle groups in the hands, such as buttoning.

Geriatrician: A physician who specializes in elder care.

Habilitation: An approach to caring for a person with a progressive dementia that focuses on validating the patient's underlying emotions, maintaining dignity, creating moments for success, and using all remaining skills. (See the list of tenets on page 7.)

Habilitator: A synonym for care partner.

Long-term-care facility: A nursing home or other community-based health care center that provides care for the remainder of a person's life.

Neuro-psych evaluation: A method of evaluating cognitive impairment, as part of the diagnostic workup for Alzheimer's disease.

Optimal independent functional level: The highest-level physical, social, and cognitive performance that can be expected, based on the patient's stage of disease and environmental factors.

Orientation: The patient's recognition of time (day, year, time, holidays), place (country, state, town, facility, address, room), self, and relationships.

Palliative care: The routine care of a patient, not designed to cure.

Plan of care: A written plan that is regularly assessed to assure that the patient's physical, social, emotional, and spiritual needs are being met *over a specific period of time.* (See page 28.)

Safe Return: A program run by the National Alzheimer's Association that helps families find patients who have wandered away. (See page 217.)

Share-care: An arrangement among care partners to take turns looking after several Alzheimer's patients for a given period of time. (See page 171.)

Special-care unit (SCU): A unit within a nursing home or other facility that cares exclusively for people with progressive dementia. (See page 189.)

Sundown syndrome or sundowning: The occurrence of problematic behavior late in the afternoon or early evening. (See page 63.)

Verbal casserole: The fragmented language expression of some late-middle-stage Alzheimer's patients, often consisting of many words in no particular order or relationship. (See page 78.)

· APPENDIX ·

Good Food for People with Alzheimer's

Staples to Have on Hand

Keep your pantry stocked with a variety of easy-to-prepare foods.
Here are some suggestions:

Canned cocktail franks
Canned fish such as tuna, salmon, and crab
Canned kidney beans, lentils, and chickpeas, to add to soups and
salads for variety and nutrition
Canned soups, including broth and creamed soups. (Add cooked
vegetables or pasta to soups for variety.) Soups provide a hearty
snack or meal any time of day.
Herbal teas
Ice cream cones (place a small marshmallow in the tip to prevent
dripping)
Juice drink boxes
Packaged bread or muffin mixes — for example, corn, banana,
date nut, and lemon poppy seed. (For easier handling of the
batter, use less milk than called for in the directions; for a but-
tery taste, use melted butter instead of oil.)
Pretzels, potato sticks, and other simple snacks
Quick flour mix, such as Bisquick, for making biscuits, pancakes,
and desserts

Rice cakes
Small boxes of dry cereal

Finger Foods

Families and professionals who oversee the dining needs of people with Alzheimer's know that finger foods are the best choice for maintaining dignity, providing opportunities for success, and encouraging proper nutrition. Such foods require no utensils, condiments, or plates, and can be served at any time of day.

Removing extra silverware, condiments, and dinnerware from the table makes dining a nonthreatening experience for the patient. The care partner's presentation of a simple food to be eaten from the hand is a positive experience for both care partner and patient.

Preparing Finger Foods

Pita bread, tortillas, and hot dog rolls are excellent "wraps" for finger foods. They are easy to see and hold, and you can easily find whole-wheat and other nutritious varieties. Ingredients for wraps can be old standbys such as tuna, egg salad, or peanut butter and jelly, or they can be more exotic (see suggestions below). For patients in later stages of the disease, all kinds of foods can be blended and used as sandwich fillings. Don't let your own sense of what is palatable interfere with preparation or serving; watch the patient's demeanor for signs of a positive eating experience. The goal is to get the patient to eat — and do so independently. Weight gain is generally not a concern. And as the patient becomes less active in later stages of the disease, she may lose weight naturally.

Nutritious Sandwich Fillings

Cottage cheese and herbs (or fruit preserves)
Cranberry sauce (sliced) with cheddar cheese
Cream cheese and fruit preserves
Cream cheese and green olives

Cream cheese and pimiento

Cream cheese with flax seeds and drained crushed pineapple

Eggs, scrambled, fried, or boiled and cut up (because eggs are difficult to see, they may be best used as a sandwich filling)

Filling from frozen pot pies

Hummus — add soft chopped vegetables (scallions, red peppers, or fresh tomato) for added flavor and attractive appearance

Mashed black or kidney beans (canned) and tomato chunks

Mashed carrots with melted cheese

Mashed potatoes with melted cheese

Meat, deboned and cut into small pieces

Mild Mexican salsa

Peanut butter (with or without jelly)

Salmon salad with raisins

Soft or hard cheeses

Spaghetti, cut up, with thick sauce

Tuna, chicken, or egg salad (soak chopped celery and/or onion for ten minutes to make it easier to chew)

Vegetable spreads

Other Finger Foods

FRUITS

Apples, pears, or peaches, peeled and cut into wedges

Banana slices with peanut butter

Dried fruit

Grapes

Pears, sliced, with soft cheese spread

Pineapple chunks

Tomatoes (grape or cherry)

VEGETABLES

Asian vegetables, such as canned baby corn, water chestnuts, or bamboo shoots, or fresh, washed sugar snap peas, snow peas, or daikon (a Japanese sweet radish)

Broccoli, carrots, cauliflower, green beans, or zucchini, cut up and parboiled for three to five minutes to make them easier to chew; drain and serve warm.

Celery filled with peanut butter or flavored cream cheese

Cucumber, sliced and spread with hummus

Dry-roasted peas (sold in health food stores)

French fries (oven-roasted)

Potato wedges or puffs

Sweet potato cubes or wedges (oven-roasted)

Vegetable loaf (use vegetables in place of meat; cut into cubes and serve cool)

Meat and Fish

Chicken nuggets

Cocktail franks wrapped in triangle or crescent rolls

Fish sticks

Meatballs (small)

Shrimp (peeled)

Turkey meatloaf (cubed and cooled)

Breakfast Foods

Bacon or sausage mixed into pancake batter, cooked, then rolled up

Boiled eggs (best served cut up in a sandwich)

Cinnamon toast strips

French toast strips made with thick bread

Nutritious dry breakfast cereals (mix with nuts or raisins, if desired, and serve without milk)

Waffles, especially whole-wheat

Lunch

Cheese cubes

Grilled cheese on dark rye, cut in quarters

Grilled scrambled egg (and bacon if desired) on dark rye, cut in quarters

Pizza cut into small squares
Ravioli or tortellini without sauce
Spring rolls or egg rolls
String cheese
Ziti or other finger-sized pasta, plain or with Parmesan cheese

DESSERTS
Animal crackers
Ginger snaps spread with cream cheese
Jell-O made with fruit yogurt instead of cold water, served in an
   ice cream cone if desired
Pudding (instant) in an ice cream cone

SNACKS
Energy bars
Goldfish crackers
Granola bars (chewy)
Popcorn
Potato sticks
Pretzels
Sesame sticks or crackers
Shelled peanuts
Soybeans
Vegetable chips

Blender Beverages

If the patient dislikes taking medication, liquid forms can be dis-
guised in beverages mixed in a blender.

Banana Nana: blend 1 cup vanilla ice cream, 1 very ripe banana,
   and 1 teaspoon vanilla.
Berry Berry: blend 1½ cups cranberry juice, 1 cup frozen blueber-
   ries, and a dash of lemon juice.

Fruit Smoothie: blend 1 cup fruit yogurt, 1 cup sorbet, and 1 cup orange juice.

Ginger Snap: blend 1 cup peach ice cream, ½ cup crushed ginger snaps, and a dash of ground ginger.

Lemon Sparkler: blend 1 cup lemon sherbet and 2 cups lemonade. Remove from blender and add 1 cup sparkling or soda water.

Maple Delight: blend 1 cup milk, 1 large scoop vanilla ice cream, 1 teaspoon molasses, 1 teaspoon maple syrup, and 1 teaspoon vanilla.

Pistachio Green Goddess: blend 2 cups pistachio ice cream, 2 cups green tea, and 1 tablespoon sugar.

Strawberry Smoothie: blend 1½ cups strawberry yogurt, 1 cup apple juice, and 1 cup strawberries.

Tomato Energizer: blend 2 cups minestrone soup, 1 cup tomato juice, 2 teaspoons lemon juice, ½ teaspoon white pepper, and 8 ice cubes.

Vanilla Pick-Me-Up: blend 1½ cups vanilla yogurt, 1 teaspoon wheat germ, 1 egg, and 2 teaspoons vanilla.

Further Resources

Organizations

Administration on Aging. This agency of the federal government publishes a useful fact sheet titled "Respite: What Caregivers Need Most." Telephone: 202-619-0724. Available on the Internet: www.aoa.gov/fact sheets/Respite.html.

AllExperts. A volunteer organization staffed with physicians, nurses, home care providers, and other experts who answer questions on-line about the disease process, nursing facilities, home care, and other issues. Only on-line services are offered: www.allexperts.com.

Alzheimer's Association. The most prominent Alzheimer's organization in the country, with chapters nationwide. It provides information, suggestions, referrals, and other support options to patients, care partners, and families. 919 North Michigan Ave., Suite 1100, Chicago, IL 60611-1676; telephone: 800-272-3900 or 312-335-8700; fax: 312-335-1110; www.alz .org.

Alzheimer's Disease Education and Referral Center (ADEAR). An affiliate of the National Institute on Aging (NIA) that offers current, comprehensive, and definitive information and resources on Alzheimer's. ADEAR Center, P.O. Box 8250, Silver Spring, MD 20907-8250; telephone: 800-438-4380; fax: 301-495-3334; www.alzheimers.org.

American Association of Homes and Services for the Aging (AAHSA). A national nonprofit organization offering information on more than 5,600 nonprofit elder-care and Alzheimer's-care facilities. 2519 Connecticut Ave. NW, Washington, DC 20008-1520; telephone: 202-783-2242; fax: 202-783-2255; www.aahsa.org.

American Association of Retired Persons. Anyone over fifty can be a member of AARP. The organization deals with many age-related issues, including living with Alzheimer's disease. It offers brochures ranging from early diagnosis to dealing with loss. AARP has offices in cities throughout the country. 601 E St. NW, Washington, DC 20049; telephone: 800-424-3410; fax: 202-434-2588; www.aarp.org.

American Bar Association Commission on Legal Problems of the Elderly. The commission offers advice on advance planning matters, including quality-of-life issues. Its publication *Consumer's Tool Kit for Health Care Advance Planning* contains a variety of self-help worksheets, suggestions, and resources designed for ease of use. 740 15th St. NW, Washington, DC 20005-1022; telephone: 202-662-8690; www.abanet.org/elderly.

American Health Care Association (AHCA). A federation of affiliated state health organizations that provides information about nursing homes and other managed-care housing options. 1201 L St. NW, Washington, DC 20005; telephone: 202-842-4444; www.ahca.org.

American Society on Aging. One of the largest professional associations on issues dealing with aging, the ASA promotes the dignity and well-being of the elderly and provides excellent information on caregiving and housing options. 833 Market St., Suite 511, San Francisco, CA 94103; telephone: 415-974-9600; www.asaging.org.

A Place for Mom. A free national elder care referral service that helps care partners locate, compare, and choose local assisted-living facilities, nursing homes, and/or Alzheimer's special-care facilities. The organization also provides help in finding long-term-care insurance and tips on visiting nursing facilities. There are representatives of the organization in every state. Telephone: 877-MOMDAD-9 (877-666-3239); www.a placeformom.com.

Assisted Living Federation of America. ALFA provides information and referrals about assisted-living facilities. 9411 Lee Hwy., Plaza Suite J, Fairfax, VA 22031; telephone: 703-691-8100; fax: 703-691-8106; www .alfa.org.

Benjamin B. Green-Field National Alzheimer's Library and Resource Center. The largest Alzheimer's library in the world. 919 North Michigan Ave., Chicago, IL 60611; telephone: 800-272-3900 or 312-335-9602; fax: 312-335-0214; www.alz.org/ResourceCenter/Programs/LibraryServices .htm.

Calhoun County Medical Care Facility and Marian E. Burch adult day care center. The Web site lists the comparative costs of adult day care and long-term or permanent nursing home stays as a basis for comparison.

1150 E. Michigan Ave., Battle Creek, MI 49014; telephone: 269-962-5458; fax: 269-962-7011; www.ccmcf.com.

California Association for Adult Day Services. Provides a list of many types of adult day care services. 921 11th St., Suite 701, Sacramento, CA 95814; telephone: 916-552-7400; fax: 916-552-7404; www.cads.org/adultday.html.

Case Management Society of America. A professional organization dedicated to the continuing education of case managers, nurses, and other health professionals and to networking around issues such as case management, social work, disease management, and rehabilitation. The organization offers helpful resources and referrals. 8201 Cantrell Rd., Suite 230, Little Rock, AR 72227; telephone: 501-225-2229; fax: 501-221-9068; www.cmsa.org.

Children of Aging Parents. CAPS is a nonprofit association that provides help in finding care-partner support groups and in locating geriatric care managers. 1609 Woodbourne Rd., Suite 302A, Levittown, PA 19057; telephone: 800-227-7294; www.caps4caregivers.org.

Cognitive Neurology and Alzheimer's Disease Center. The center provides information and support to the Alzheimer's sufferer and care partner, including reports on the latest research. 320 East Superior St., Searle 11-450, Chicago, IL 60611-3008; telephone: 312-908-9339; www.brain.nwu.edu/.

Eldercare Locator. A service of the U.S. Administration on Aging. Nationwide toll-free service helps find local services for older people. Telephone: 800-677-1116; www.eldercare.gov.

ElderCare Online. An Internet-based resource committed to helping Alzheimer's and dementia care partners find support and understanding, as well as educational resources and information. 54 Amuxen Ct., Islip, NY 11751; www.alzwell.com.

Family Caregiver Alliance. A nonprofit organization that focuses on helping home care partners by supplying many publications and much useful information. The magazine *Today's Caregiver,* available in print or online, has special Alzheimer's sections. A subscription includes a free weekly e-mail newsletter; for subscription information, call 800-829-2734. 690 Market St., Suite 600, San Francisco, CA 94104; telephone: 415-434-3388; fax: 415-434-3508; www.caregiver.org.

Fisher Center for Alzheimer's Research Foundation. An on-line site provides information and links on elder care, care-partner and patient resources, and up-to-date information on Alzheimer's research. One Intrepid Square, West 46th St. and 12th Ave., New York, NY 10036; telephone: 800-ALZ-INFO (259-4636); www.alzinfo.org.

Hospice Foundation of America. With a national database of hospice providers, the foundation offers help in finding the right hospice. 2001 S St. NW, Suite 300, Washington, DC 20009; telephone: 800-854-3402; fax: 202-638-5312; www.hospicefoundation.org.

Information Source for Adult Day Centers. Provides an extensive list of state associations and other contacts as well as information for operators of adult day care centers. 5220 Beckwyck Dr., Fuquay-Varina, NC 27526; telephone: 919-552-0254; fax: 919-552-0155; www.theinfosource 4adc.com/Links.html.

Law and Aging Resource Guide. The American Bar Association publishes this state-by-state directory of legal resources and services available for seniors. 740 15th St. NW, Washington, DC 20005-1022; telephone: 202-662-8690; www.abanet.org.

Medicare Rights Center (MRC). An information resource on Medicare coverage. 1460 Broadway, 17th Fl., New York, NY 10036; telephone: 212-869-3850; fax: 212-869-3532; www.medicarerights.org.

Metropolitan Area Agency on Aging of Minneapolis/St. Paul. Provides a checklist for assessing day care centers. 1600 University Ave. West, Suite 300, St. Paul, MN 55104; telephone: 651-641-8612; fax: 651-641-8618; www.tcaging.org/com_adck.htm.

National Academy of Elder Law Attorneys. NAELA offers an on-line database of its member attorneys by location. 1604 N. Country Club Rd., Tucson, AZ 85716; telephone: 520 881 4005; www.naela.com/naela/resources.htm.

National Adult Day Services Association. NADSA offers information, standards, and referrals on many adult day care programs. 8201 Greensboro Drive, Suite 300, McLean, VA 22102; telephone: 866-890-7357 or 703-610-9035; fax: 703-610-9005; www.nadsa.org.

National Association for Continence (NAFC). An incontinence resource. P.O. Box 8310, Spartanburg, SC 29305; telephone: 800-BLADDER (252-3337) or 864-579-7900; fax: 864-579-7902; www.nafc.org.

National Association of Area Agencies on Aging (N4A). This umbrella organization for almost nine hundred area agencies on aging functions as a clearinghouse for information for elders and care partners seeking local support resources. Information is available in English and Spanish. 927 15th St. NW, 6th Fl., Washington, DC 20005; telephone: 202-296-8130; fax: 202-296-8134; www.n4a.org.

National Association for Home Care and Hospice (NAHC). Provides more than 22,000 resources for those seeking hospice or home care. The publication *How to Choose a Home Care Provider,* available on-line or in print, tells how to select the right provider and what to do if something goes wrong, and explains standard billing practices. 228 Seventh St. SE, Washington, DC 20003; telephone: 202-547-7424; fax: 202-547-3540; www.nahc.com.

National Caregiving Foundation. Produces the Caregivers Support Kit, which is designed to address every aspect of care partnering and simplify daily tasks. 891 N. Pitt St., Alexandria, VA 22314-1765; telephone: 800-930-1357; www.caregivingfoundation.org.

National Citizens Coalition for Nursing Home Reform (NCCHR). Provides useful information and referrals to nursing homes. 1424 16th St. NW, Suite 202, Washington, DC 20002; telephone: 202-332-2275; fax: 202-332-2949; www.ncchr.org.

National Consumer Law Center, Seniors Initiative (NCLC). Focuses on consumer issues, including bankruptcy, foreclosures, misrepresentation, fraud, and predatory sales practices. Publishes newsletters such as *Avoiding Living Will Scams, Medical Debt and Seniors: How Consumer Laws Can Help*, and *When You Can't Go Home Again: Using Consumer Law to Protect Nursing Facility Residents*. 1629 K St. NW, Suite 600, Washington, DC 20006; telephone: 202-986-6060; www.nclc.org/initiatives/ seniors_initiative/index.shtml.

National Council on Aging (NCOA). The council is concerned with the "dignity, self-determination, well-being, and contributions" of elders. Brochures include *Alzheimer's Patient Guide* and *Alzheimer's Caregiver Guide*. 409 Third St. SW, Suite 200, Washington, DC 20024; telephone: 202-479-1200; TTD: 202-479-6674; fax: 202-479-0735; www .ncoa.org.

National Hospice and Palliative Care Organization (NHPCO). Offers several brochures about hospice and palliative care. 1700 Diagonal Rd., Suite 300, Alexandria, VA 22314; telephone: 800-646-6460 or 703-837-1500; fax: 703-525-5762; www.nhpco.org.

National Institute on Aging (NIA). This division of NIH offers a great resource directory, with information on the latest research and clinical studies, including state and federal agencies and resource centers. Bldg. 31, Rm. 5C27, 31 Center Dr., MSC 2292, Bethesda, MD 20892; telephone: 301-496-1752; www.nih.gov/nia.

National Institutes of Health (NIH). This national clearinghouse of health information helps to direct national research priorities. It is particularly helpful on disorders related to Alzheimer's. 9000 Rockville Pike, Bethesda, MD 20892; telephone: 800-438-4380; TTD: 800-222-4225; www.nih.gov.

New Lifestyles Online. A searchable state-by-state on-line database of Alzheimer's care, assisted-living, and nursing home facilities, with links to each facility. A free paper version covers housing resources in more than forty metropolitan areas. www.newlifestyles.com.

Ronald and Nancy Reagan Research Institute. The institute funds research grants to find the causes of and possible cures for Alzheimer's disease. Contact the National Alzheimer's Association for more information. Telephone: 800-272-3900; www.alz.org/researchers/reaganresearch/overview.htm.

Safe Return Program. Each individual registered in this program, sponsored by the Alzheimer's Association, receives a unique ID number imprinted on a bracelet, making it easier for law enforcement officials and others to identify the wanderer and make sure he is safely returned home. There is a one-time registration fee of $40. Contact the Alzheimer's Association Helpline: 800-660-1993.

SeniorResource.com. Offers information, support, and resources for care partners, including financial advice, humor, and a state-by-state list of resources. P.O. Box 781, Del Mar, CA 92014-0781; telephone: 858-793-7901 or 877-793-7901; fax: 858-792-9080; www.seniorresource.com.

United Seniors Health Cooperative (USHC). Nonprofit national organization committed to education and advocacy for care providers. Publications include *Long Term Care Planning: A Dollar and Sense Guide* and *Medicare Health Plan Choices: Consumer Update* (updated every January). 409 Third St. SW, Suite 200, Washington, DC 20024-3212; telephone: 202-479-6973; www.unitedseniorshealth.org.

Books

Antonangeli, Judy. *Of Two Minds.* Fidelity Press, 1995. Discusses the connection between Down's syndrome and Alzheimer's.

Brawley, Elizabeth C. *Designing for Alzheimer's Disease: Strategies for Creating a Better Care Environment.* John Wiley and Sons, 1997. A thorough approach to designing a therapeutic and safe setting for the Alzheimer's patient.

Brennan, Tim. Through His Eyes: The Collective Works of Tim Brennan. Brennan, diagnosed with Alzheimer's in November 1993, immediately began keeping an on-line journal providing a firsthand patient's perspective. www .nhisgarden.com/his_eyes/page_index.html.

Calkins, Margaret. *Creating Successful Dementia Care Settings,* 4 vols. Health Professions Press, 2000. A holistic and complementary approach to designing or redesigning a dementia-care facility that addresses the physical environment, staff care practices, and residents' needs.

Castleman, Michael, Dolores Gallagher-Thompson, and Matthew Naythons. *There's Still a Person in There: The Complete Guide to Treating and Coping with Alzheimer's.* Berkley, 2000. A practical approach to Alzheimer's disease, with solid information on financial planning and other issues.

Charlap, Dr. Steven S. *Making Sense of Nursing Homes: A Guide for Families.* Age Sense, 2002. Advice on financial issues, emotional support, and nonprofit and governmental resources. To order, call 866-333-5736.

Davies, Helen D., and Michael P. Jensen, *Alzheimer's: The Answers You Need.* Elder Books, 1998. For the newly diagnosed, question-and-answer sections, plus tips for coping, preparing for the future, and ameliorating the personal environment.

De Baggio, Thomas. *Losing My Mind.* Free Press, 2002. One man's inspiring attempt to stay in touch with his world as he battles Alzheimer's disease.

Fazio, Sam, Dorothy Seman, and Jane Stansell. *Rethinking Alzheimer's Care.* Health Professions Press, 1999. Although written for professional caregivers, the book underscores the need to look at the positive aspects of caring for Alzheimer's patients.

Feil, N., and V. Klerk-Rubin. *The Validation Breakthrough: Simple Techniques for Communicating with People with Alzheimer's-Type Dementia.* Health Professions Press, 2002. Simple methods for improving communication.

Glickstein, J. *Therapeutic Interventions in Alzheimer's Disease: A Program of Functional Skills for Activities of Daily Living and Communication.* Aspen Publishers, 1997. A wide range of therapeutic activities designed to stimulate the dementia patient.

Hodgson, Harriet. *Alzheimer's: Finding the Words: A Communication Guide for Those Who Care.* John Wiley and Sons, 1995. A guide for communicating with the Alzheimer's patient plus support tips for the care partner.

Kuhn, Daniel. *Alzheimer's Early Stages: First Steps in Caring and Treatment.* Hunter House, 1999. Addresses the issues many care partners face with a patient in the first stages of the disease.

Landay, David S. *Be Prepared: The Complete Financial, Legal, and Practical Guide for Living with a Life-Challenging Condition.* St. Martin's, 1999. The financial and legal challenges of living with chronic illness.

Mace, Nancy L., and Peter V. Rabins. *The 36-Hour Day.* Johns Hopkins Press, 2001. Newly reprinted, this valuable resource for the family and care partners provides comprehensive information on caring for a person with Alzheimer's disease.

Mahoney, Ellen K., Ladislav Volicer, and Ann C. Hurley. *Management of*

Challenging Behaviors in Dementia. Health Professions Press, 2000. An easy-to-understand presentation of modern scientific understanding of disruptive behavior in people suffering with dementia, with care strategies for nursing and health professionals.

McGowan, Diana Friel. *Living in the Labyrinth: A Personal Journey Through the Maze of Alzheimer's.* Delta, 1994. A first-person account of life with Alzheimer's.

Medina, John J. *What You Need to Know about Alzheimer's.* New Harbinger Publishers, 1999. Explains the biological process of the disease and considers the emotional, material, and coping issues.

National Alzheimer's Association. *Activity Programming for Persons with Dementia: A Sourcebook.* National Alzheimer's Association, 1995. How to help the Alzheimer's patient develop, enhance, and maintain relationships.

———. *Can-Do Activities for Adults with Alzheimer's Disease: Strength-Based Communication and Programming.* National Alzheimer's Association, 2001. Activities to strengthen communication skills. Available from the Benjamin B. Green-Field Library and Resource Center (catalog no. WM 450 E36 2001). Contact the Alzheimer's Association by telephone: 800-272-3900; or fax: 312-335-0214.

———. *Steps to Enhancing Communications: Interacting with Persons with Alzheimer's Disease.* National Alzheimer's Association, 1997. Tips to improve communication between the Alzheimer's patient and care partner. Single copies of the brochure are free. Available from the Benjamin B. Green-Field Library and Resource Center (catalog no. ED310Z). Contact the Alzheimer's Association by telephone: 800-272-3900; or fax: 312-335-0214.

Nissenboim, Sylvia, and Christine Vroman. *The Positive Interaction Program of Activities for People with Alzheimer's Disease.* Health Professions Press, 1998. The benefits of an active life for Alzheimer's patients.

Pierce, Charles. *Hard to Forget.* Random House, 1999. The author faces his own destiny in this memorable trip through familial Alzheimer's with humor and pathos.

Rau, Marie. *Coping with Communication Challenges in Alzheimer's Disease.* Singular Publishing Group, 1993. Improving the communications skills of the patient and care partner.

Ray, B. J. *Alzheimer's Activities: Hundreds of Activities for Men and Women with Alzheimer's Disease and Related Disorders.* Rayve Productions, 2001.

Rose, Larry. *Show Me the Way to Go Home.* Elder Books, 1996. A firsthand account by a man coping with early-onset Alzheimer's.

Schacter, Daniel L. *The Seven Sins of Memory.* Houghton Mifflin, 2001.

How the mind forgets and remembers — a new look at our brains through fascinating stories and scientific findings.

Snyder, Lisa. *Speaking Our Minds: Personal Reflections from Individuals with Alzheimer's*. W. H. Freeman, 1999. Seven Alzheimer's patients discuss their coping strategies, augmented by the author's experiences as a caregiver.

Souren, Liduin, and Emile Franssen. *Broken Connections*. Swets and Zeitlinger, 1994. Elaborates on the different levels of assistance necessary as Alzheimer's progresses.

Strauss, Claudia. *Talking to Alzheimer's: Simple Ways to Connect When You Visit with a Family Member or Friend*. New Harbinger Press, 2002. Advice on getting the most out of visiting a friend or loved one in an extended-care facility.

Visiting Nurses Association of America. *Caregiver's Handbook: A Complete Guide to Home Health Care by the Visiting Nurses Association of America*. DK Publishers, 1998. Designed to help the care partner cope with the patient's emotional and physical needs. An excellent introduction for the home care provider.

Werner, Anne P., and James Firman. *Home Care for Older People: A Consumer's Guide*. United Seniors Health Cooperative, 1994. Provides information and sample worksheets for choosing a home care provider, writing an employment contract, and solving problems related to home care. Large-print format. Available through the United Seniors Health Cooperative, 1331 H St. NW, Washington, DC 20005-4706; telephone: 202-393-6222.

Zgola, Jitka, and Gilbert Ordillon. *Bon Appétit! The Joy of Dining in Long-Term Care*. Health Professions Press, 2001. How to make mealtimes in a long-term-care facility more enjoyable and rewarding for the patient. Much of the information is also applicable to care in the home.

Videos

Alzheimer's Disease: Natural Feeding Techniques (one videocassette, 14 minutes). U.S. Veterans' Administration. Helps care partners working with patients who have feeding difficulties. Available from the U.S. Department of Commerce, National Technical Information Service, Springfield, VA 22161; telephone: 703-605-6000; www.ntis.gov/products/pages/caps_alzheimers.asp.

Alzheimer's: Is There Hope? WLIW Productions, originally aired on public television stations on November 1, 2002. Presents the researchers engaged in the scientific exploration of Alzheimer's and offers accounts of care partners. To order a copy, call 800-847-7793 or visit www.wliw.org/productions/alzh.html.

Breakfast Club: Enhancing the Communication Ability of Alzheimer's Patients (one videocassette, 25 minutes). Speech Bin, Vero Beach, FL, 1997. Examines the Breakfast Club Program, a method of easing communication for people with Alzheimer's. Available from the Benjamin B. Green-Field Library and Resource Center (catalog no. WL340 VC #717 1997).

Communicating with Older Adults and People with Dementia (one videocassette, 42 minutes). Assisted Living Best Practices, 1999. How to communicate with the memory-impaired. Experts share their knowledge of agnosia, amnesia, aphasia, apraxia, and attention deficit in persons with dementia. To order, contact Assisted Living, 4101 International Parkway, Carrollton, TX 75007; telephone: 888-578-8394.

Communication, the Heart of the Matter: The Sandwich Generation, Coping with Aging Parents (one videocassette, 20 minutes). Aquarius Health Care, Sherborn, MA, 1999. Communication concerns for care partners and caring for a loved one from a distance. Available from the Benjamin B. Green-Field Library and Resource Center (catalog no. HV 1461 VC #596 1999).

Communication: How to Communicate with Someone Who Has Alzheimer's Disease or Related Dementia (two videocassettes, 58 minutes). Healing Arts Communication, 2001. Covers a range of communication and language techniques useful in such situations as repetitive and difficult questioning, chores, aggression, and more. Available from the Benjamin B. Green-Field Library and Resource Center (catalog no. WV 270 #580 1999)

How to Have a Meaningful Visit with Your Loved One at a Nursing Facility (one videocassette, 38 minutes). Terra Nova Films, Chicago, IL, 1997. For individuals who have recently placed a loved one in a nursing facility, this film is intended to alleviate the guilt, sadness, and discomfort of visiting. Available from the Benjamin B. Green-Field Library and Resource Center (catalog no. WX 27 VC #568 1997).

Interacting with Alzheimer Patients: Tips for Family and Friends: Alzheimer Disease Do's and Don'ts (one videocassette, 20 minutes). Video Press, University of Maryland School of Medicine, Baltimore, MD, 2000. Expert Peter Rabins discusses techniques for interacting with Alzheimer's patients, including distractions, reinforcement, repetition, and independence. Available from the Benjamin B. Green-Field Library and Resource Center (catalog no. WX 27 #720 2000).

Living with Alzheimer's (three-part series on three videocassettes). Long

Island (N.Y.) Alzheimer's Foundation, 2000. Useful information and support for the care partner or health care provider. Nominated for the 2000 Telly Award. To order, contact Long Island Alzheimer's Foundation, 5 Channel Dr., Port Washington, NY 11050; telephone: 866-789-5423; www.liaf.org.

Recognizing and Responding to Emotion in Persons with Dementia (one videocassette, 26 minutes). Philadelphia Geriatric Center, Philadelphia, PA, 1997. People with dementia still have emotions and preferences even though they can no longer express their likes and dislikes. Available from the Benjamin B. Green-Field Library and Resource Center (catalog no. WY 160 VC #488 1997).

Someone I Love Has Alzheimer's (one videocassette, 17 minutes). Fanlight Productions, 1993. Filmed in a support group of children who live with a loved one with Alzheimer's. The children discuss their feelings, share ideas and issues, and offer advice to other children in their situation. Available from the Alzheimer's Association of Massachusetts, 36 Cameron Ave., Cambridge, MA 02140; telephone: 800-548-2111.

STB Forever Young video series. STB Productions. Videos with uninterrupted music to aid in relaxation and recall, designed specifically for Alzheimer's patients. Videos include "A Celebration of the Four Seasons," with Handel's *Water Music;* "Gardens, Blossoms, and Blooms," a virtual walk through a beautiful garden with gentle breezes, waterfall, and singing birds; "Christmas Hearth," a holiday theme with a crackling fire; and "County Fair Memories," featuring ragtime music and the sights, feel, and flavor of an old-time county fair. Other titles also available. To order, contact STB Productions, 71 Rinewalt St., Williamsville, NY 14221; telephone: 716-626-5319; www.stbvideo.com.

Untitled video on communication (one videocassette, 20 minutes). National Alzheimer's Association, Chicago, 1990. Care partners describe their challenges and solutions for communicating with the patient. Ways to help care partners and patients express their thoughts. Available from the Benjamin B. Green-Field Library and Resource Center (catalog no. WM 220 VC #248 1990).

Music and Old-Time Radio

CD Universe. A large selection of nostalgia and oldies' music and spoken-word CDs, audiocassettes, DVDs, and videotapes. www.cduniverse.com.

Radio Spirits. Boxed sets of VHS, CD, and audiocassettes of old radio broadcasts, including Bob Hope, Jack Benny, the Lone Ranger, Nero

Wolfe, the Shadow, and much more. P.O. Box 3107, Wallingford, CT 06492; telephone: 203-265-8044; www.radiospirits.com.

Tower Records. Stores across the country and around the world carry thousands of CDs, LPs, and cassettes of oldies and classics. www.tower records.com.

Wireless Catalog from the NPR Shop (operated by National Public Radio). Audio and videotapes of classic radio and TV shows. Telephone: 800-669-9999; www.shop.npr.org.

Products

Adaptations by Adrian. Clothing specially designed for the wheelchair-bound. Men's and women's clothing from undergarments to outerwear. P.O. Box 65, San Marcos, CA 92079-0065; telephone: 800-831-2577; www .adrianscloset.com.

AliMed. AliMed Wander Alarm and hundreds of home help aids, including security, kitchen, and bath aids, bedside motion detectors, and bed alarms. 297 High St., Dedham, MA 02026; telephone: 800-225-2610; www.alimed.com.

Allegro Medical Supply. Bathroom security/assistance and other elder-care products, with savings on bulk purchases of incontinence products. Telephone: 800-861-3211; www.allegromedical.com.

Alzheimer's Store. Products for patient and care partner needs, including security, dressing, incontinence aids, and activities, with many stage-specific products. On-line or free print catalog available. Alzheimer's Store Ageless Design, Inc., 12633 159th Ct., North Jupiter, FL 33478-6669; telephone: 800-752-3238; www.alzstore.com.

A-Med Care Center. Incontinence, safety, bathroom, and skin-care products. Many samples available. 800-552-2633; www.a-med.com.

American Ramp Systems. Portable and permanent wheelchair ramps for sale or rent; free in-home evaluations anywhere in the United States. Especially helpful for middle-stage or late-stage patients. 202 West First St., Boston, MA 02127-1110; telephone: 800-649-5215; www.american ramp.com.

Ameriphone. Communication devices, including videophones, enhanced-audio phones, auto-dialing phones, and voice-activated phones. 12082 Western Ave., Garden Grove, CA 92841-2913; telephone: 800-874-3005; TTY: 800-772-2889; www.ameriphone.com.

Assisted Living Store. Home modifications for the elderly and people with disabilities as well as products relating to incontinence, security, bed and bath modification, dining, and dressing. 7687 Hyde Ave., South Cottage Grove, MN 55016; telephone: 888-388-5862; www.assistedliving store.com.

Beyond Barriers. Products for home modification, including bath, toileting, kitchen, and general house use (faucets, auto-flush toilets, grab handles, etc.). Access One, Inc., 25679 Gramford Ave., Wyoming, MN 55092; telephone: 800-561-2223; www.beyondbarriers.com.

Buck and Buck Designs. Fashion wear for people with disabilities, with special items for Alzheimer's patients. Very large selection of men's and women's styles. Buck and Buck, Inc., 3111 27th Ave., South Seattle, WA 98144-6502; telephone: 800-458-0600; www.buckandbuck.com.

Care Medical Equipment. Incontinence and security products, bathroom aids. Free catalog. 1877 NE Seventh Ave., Portland, OR 97212; telephone: 800-443-7091; www.blvd.com/carecatalog.

Care Trak, Inc. Many different kinds of alerts and systems to help prevent wandering or track the wanderer, including GPS positioning devices, waterproof transmitters, and invisible perimeter systems. 1031 Autumn Ridge Rd., Carbondale, IL 62901-9745; telephone: 800-842-4537; www .caretrak.com.

Caregiving Solutions.com. Products for patients in all stages of the disease, ranging from doorknob covers and door entry barriers to bathing/ toileting accessories and gentle personal cleansing products like tearless shampoo. Advice and news about Alzheimer's are offered on the Web site. Alzheimer Solutions, 3122 Knorr St., Philadelphia, PA 19149; telephone: 215-624-2098; www.caregiving-solutions.com.

Clothing Solutions. For women, dresses, muumuus, dusters, two-piece sets, blouses, pants, fleece and other warmer clothing, footwear, sleepwear, and underwear; for men, dressy and casual wear, fleece and warmer clothing, footwear, sleepwear, and underwear, all designed to make dressing easier for the care provider and patient. 1525 West Alton Ave., Santa Ana, CA 92704; telephone: 800-336-2660; www.specialclothing .com.

Colonial Medical Assisted Devices. Door monitors, banner door alarms, exit alerts, knob guards, personal urine alarms, pressure-sensitive alarm mats, and other security devices. 14 Celina Ave. #15, Nashua, NH 03063; telephone: 800-323-6794; colonialmedical.com.

Comfort Clothing. A full line of men's and women's clothing for the special needs of Alzheimer's patients, from underwear to Polartec fleece. Telephone: 888-640-0814; www.comfortclothing.com.

Control Products. Thermostat regulator with auto-call. Telephone: 800-947-9098.

Digital Angel. Electronic tracking devices. With GPS technology, the Alzheimer's patient can be tracked anywhere in the world to within seventy-five feet. The wristband transmitter signals a fall or a dramatic change in temperature around the wearer, and the wanderer alert automatically signals when the wearer goes beyond preset boundaries. South St. Paul, MN; telephone: 866-DGTL-ANGL (348-5264); www.digital angel.net.

Dr. Leonard's. Velcro-closing shoes and other easy-to-wear footwear, plus other home health aids. P.O. Box 7821, Edison, NJ 08818-7821; telephone: 800-785-0880; www.drleonards.com.

Elder Corner. Bathroom aids like full-tub safety mats and tub safety bars, dressing accessories (coiler shoelaces that don't need to be tied), kitchen aids (large-handled flatware), personal care accessories (ergonomically correct bed and back pillows), and more. Telephone: 888-777-1816; www.elder corner.com.

Elder Store. Beamer Video Phone, waterproof sheeting, bed rails, and other elder-care aids and accessories. 920 Park Lane Ct., Alpharetta, GA 30022-2623; telephone: 888-833-8875; www.elderstore.net.

Exclusively Seniors. Home health care products, including bedding protection and incontinence, bathroom safety, back, neck, and foot therapy aids. Telephone: 866-477-7778; www.exclusivelyseniors.com.

Express Medical Supply. Many incontinence products and other medical supplies. On-line or free print catalog available. 218 Seebold, Spur Fenton, MO 63026; telephone: 800-633-2139; www.exmed.net.

Eyes on Elders. Medication dispensers and reminders, fall-detection devices that work even when user is disoriented, unconscious, or otherwise unable to call for help, and remote video-monitoring systems. Featured on MSNBC. VisionAge Technologies, LLC, P.O. Box 231202, Encinitas, CA 92023-1202; telephone: 877-460-5578; www.eyesonelders.com.

Fashions for Special Needs. Adaptive clothing, including wheelchair ponchos, unisex jeans, incontinence clothing, nightwear, wraps, and all-weather gear. 8251 Ridge Rd., RR 4, Welland, ON, Canada L3B 5N7; telephone: 905-384-0741; www.specialneedsclothing.com.

Five Wishes Living Will. This is the most personalized and comprehensive living will, addressing personal, emotional, and spiritual needs as well as medical wishes. It is recognized as a viable document in thirty-five states. Easy to fill out. Aging with Dignity, P.O. Box 1661, Tallahassee, FL 32302; telephone: 888-5WISHES (594-7437); www.agingwithdig nity.org.

Geriatric Resources. Stage-specific products for the care partner and patient, from aromatherapy workbooks to doorstops. Many sensory stimulation products are offered, as well as products designed for professional caregivers. Several catalogs to choose from. Geriatric Resources, Inc., P.O. Box 239, Radium Springs, NM 88054; telephone: 800-359-0390; www.geriatric-resources.com.

Home Delivery Incontinent Supplies. Web-based or mail-order home delivery of a large selection of incontinence products. 9385 Dielman Industrial Dr., Olivette, MO 63132; telephone: 800-2MY-HOME (269-4663); www.hdis.com.

Home Remedies. Automated medication dispensers. Telephone: 800-908-0907.

International Environmental Solutions: Automatic shut-off faucets. 2830 Scherer Dr. N, Suite 310, St. Petersburg, FL 33716; telephone: 800-972-8348; www.ezflo.com.

Internet Wallpaper Store. More than two hundred murals that can be used to camouflage doorways or windows. Telephone: 877-255-0907; www .wallpaperstore.com.

J. C. Penney Special Needs Catalog. Adaptive clothing and home assisting devices. P.O. Box 2021, Milwaukee, WI 53201-2021; telephone: 800-222-6161.

Life at Home. Devices to make the home safe, including wireless and silent wanderer alarms (so the patient isn't frightened), automatic stovetop fire stoppers, carbon monoxide alarms, bathtub grips, doorknob covers, appliance latches, and electronic pill reminders/dispensers. 3630-F Trousdale Dr., Nashville, TN 37204; telephone: 800-653-1923; www.life home.com.

Maddak, Inc., Ableware. Products for independent and assisted living, including bathroom, kitchen, security, communication, tactile/exercise, and therapeutic/recreational aids. 661 Rte. 23, South Wayne, NJ 07470; telephone: 973-628-7600; www.maddak.com.

Maxi Aids. Devices and aids for assisted living and home care, including folding shower chairs, tub and shower mats, no-spill urinals, grab bars and hand grips, toileting aids, and tieless shoelaces. 42 Executive Blvd., Farmingdale, NY 11735; telephone: 800-522-6294; www.maxiaids .com.

MedicAlert. A bracelet or pendant bearing the internationally recognized symbol offers protection for Alzheimer's patients with allergies and other medical problems by alerting any care provider to the wearer's special needs. MedicAlert Foundation International, 2323 Colorado Ave., Turlock, CA 95382; telephone: 800-432-5378; www.medicalert.org.

North Coast Medical Supply. The Functional Solutions catalog features a wide variety of products, including dressing aids, household helpers, adaptive eating utensils, exercise equipment, and transfer devices. 18305

Sutter Blvd., Morgan Hill, CA 95037-2845; telephone: 800-235-7054; www.ncmedical.com.

Personal Touch Health Care Supply. Specialty clothing, including dresses, pants, sweaters and sweatshirts, footwear, and slacks for men and women with incontinence, mobility, and coordination issues. Free shipping on on-line orders of $100 or more. P.O. Box 230321, Brooklyn, NY 11223; telephone: 888-626-1703; www.adaptiveapparel.com.

Pro-Active Eldercare. The themes of the Alzheimer's Survival Kits, which include dozens of activities, range from Springtime to Quilting to Spiritual to Cooking to suit the interests of each Alzheimer's patient. P.O. Box 355, Littleton, MA 01460; telephone: 866-447-0009; fax: 866-447-0008; www.proactiveeldercare.com.

Pyro-Control. Automatic fire-extinguishing system for the stovetop. Telephone: 888-616-7976.

Quilts by Mémère. Handcrafted quilts, bibs, and clothing protectors for adults. www.quiltsbymemere.

Safe and Sound. Safety aids and equipment for seniors, including antiscald valves, large-handled utensils, tub bars and bathtub rails, antislip tub and shower mats, hand-held shower valves, and carbon monoxide alarms. 2490 General Armistead Ave., Suite 202, Norristown, PA 19403; telephone: 610-539-7020; www.123safe.com.

Sammons Preston. Security, bed and bath, home care, adaptive dinnerware, and other aids designed for disabled or cognitively impaired people. Offices in the U.S. and Canada. 4 Sammons Ct., Bolingbrook, IL 60440; telephone: 800-323-5547; www.sammonspreston.com.

Sands Healthcare. Craft project kits. Catalogs include Primelife (for the elderly), Christian Activities, and Judaic Activities. P.O. Box 513, 75 Mill St., Colchester, CT 06415; telephone: 800-243-9232; www.ssww.com.

Security World. Security equipment, including motion detectors, personal alarms, and doorknob alarms. Telephone: 800-669-7328; www.security world.com.

SeniorClix. Adaptive clothing, elder-care products, and the *Sing Along with Barbara* VHS video series, which features seniors singing and interacting in an elder-care setting accompanied on the piano by their exuberant music teacher. 1218 3rd Ave., Suite 500, Seattle, WA 98101; telephone: 1-800-448-5213; www.seniorclix.com.

Seniors, Inc. Adaptive clothing for men and women, including many duster styles, flounces, pantsuits, polo shirts, and jogging suits. 1225 Wagner Dr., P.O. Box 1817, Albertville, AL 35950; telephone: 800-524-4677; www.seniorsinc.com.

Silvert's Elderly Care Clothing. Men's and women's clothing for people with special needs. Free catalog available. Telephone: 1-800-387-7088; www.silverts.com.

Specialty Care Shoppe. Clothing for people with special needs, including those with continence problems, "undressers," those with limited mobility, and Alzheimer's patients in all stages. 16126 E. 161st St. S, Bixby, OK 74008; telephone: 918-366-1208; www.specialtycareshoppe.com.

Stupell Industries. Many styles of faux windows to replace a mirror with a soothing scene. 14 Industrial La., Johnston, RI 02919; telephone: 401-831-5640; www.stupellind.com.

Talon Clothing. Adaptive clothing, including rain gear and outdoor gear such as fleece and water/windproof items, many suited for wheelchair use. 1840 160th St., Suite 247, Surrey, BC, Canada V4A 4X4; www.talon clothing.com.

Telko. Chiming motion detector. Telephone: 800-888-3556.

Trader Joe's. Many finger foods. Stores in eighteen states. Telephone: 800-746-7857; www.traderjoes.com.

Wallpaper Store. Hundreds of murals that can be used to camouflage doors. TandB Decorators, P.O. Box 211, Port Monmouth, NJ 07758; telephone: 800-473-1303; www.thewallpaperstore.com.

WanderCare. Tracking/alert system can track the wanderer from up to a mile away, call the caregiver when the wanderer has strayed, and provide constant updates on the wanderer's location and activity. Telephone: 516-334-7187; www.scorpion-security.com.

Index